T0380723

Note: None of the photographs of Larry were altered or modified to enhance his physique or appearence.

21st Century Fitness®

What will happen NEXT is worth telling NOW.

In my 75th year, I am blessed to have acquired the 8 essentials of youth.

Larry Nachman

Dedication

To my 21st Century Fitness students in Greenville, Landrum and Charleston, South Carolina.

If not for you, I would have never had the nerve to step up to the plate and produce this book.

Mission

To inspire men and women of all ages in search of the elusive Fountain of Youth.

To display visual proof—living proof—that we can retain the essentials of youth at 75 and over.

To share the fact that we can preserve the physical joys of youth longer than people have previously believed possible.

To introduce a new standard of anatomical excellence in physical well-being.

Introduction

Everyone realizes no easy solution exists to fight the aging process and believes getting "old" is inevitable.

People know factors exist that supposedly maintain youth, but which ones actually work remains a mystery.

Some say genetics.
Some say nutrition.
Some say exercise.
Some say attitude.

All are correct. Each is a piece of the puzzle.

More importantly, though, the process of assembling these pieces is an art. There is a tapestry to be woven, using these pieces, to complete the design.

This book offers visual proof that we can be young at 75 and over, as well as what it can look like. The Fountain of Youth, fabled since the time of Ponce de León, is now a reality.

Larry Nachman May, 2009

21st Century Fitness®
Sleek, lean, flexible, agile & toned.

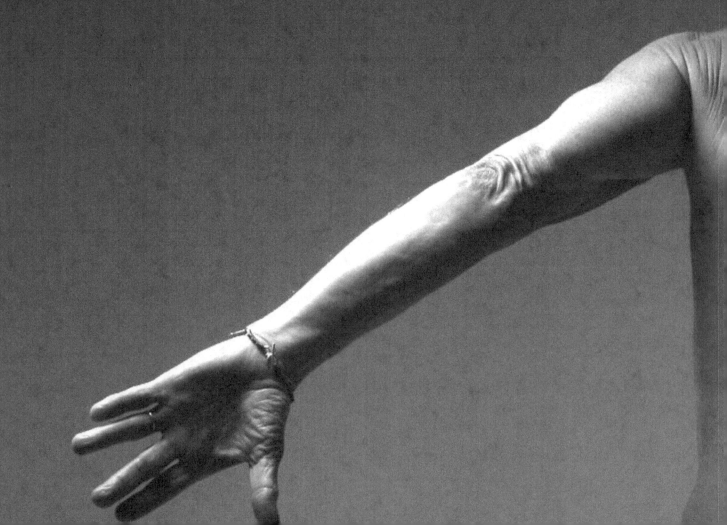

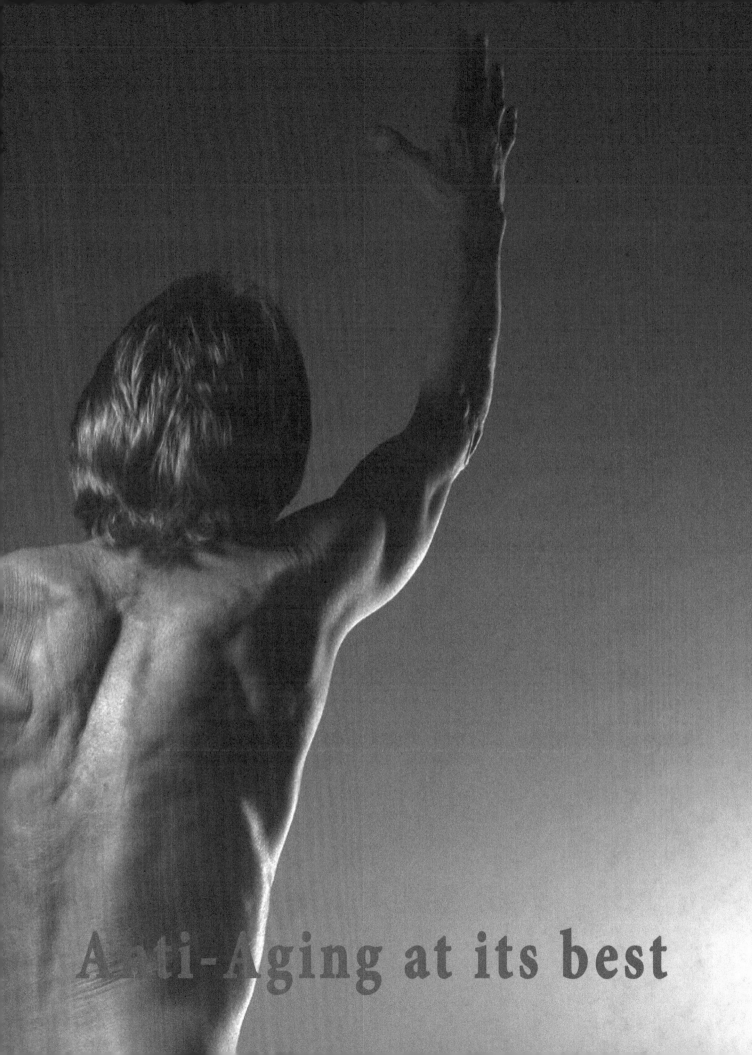

Anti-Aging at its best

The **FIRST** evidence-based formula of exercise & nutrition for staying young or returning to youth.

From the universe of fitness regimens: Larry tested, edited, rejected and refined to create a formula of exercise and nutrition that allowed him to become living proof that one can have all 8 essentials of youth at 75 and over.

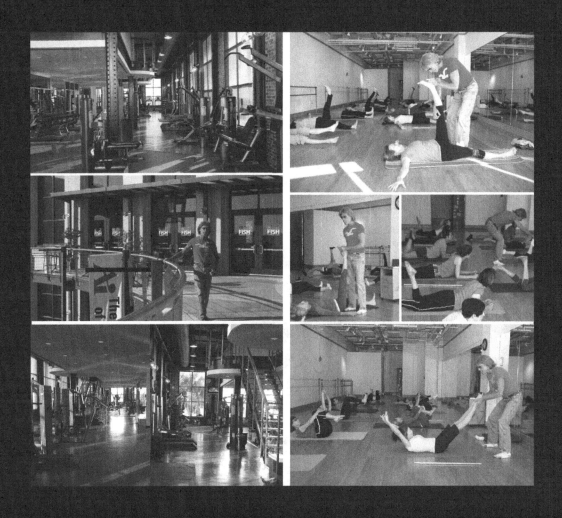

21st Century Fitness

The New Standard of Anatomical Excellence in the World of Fitness

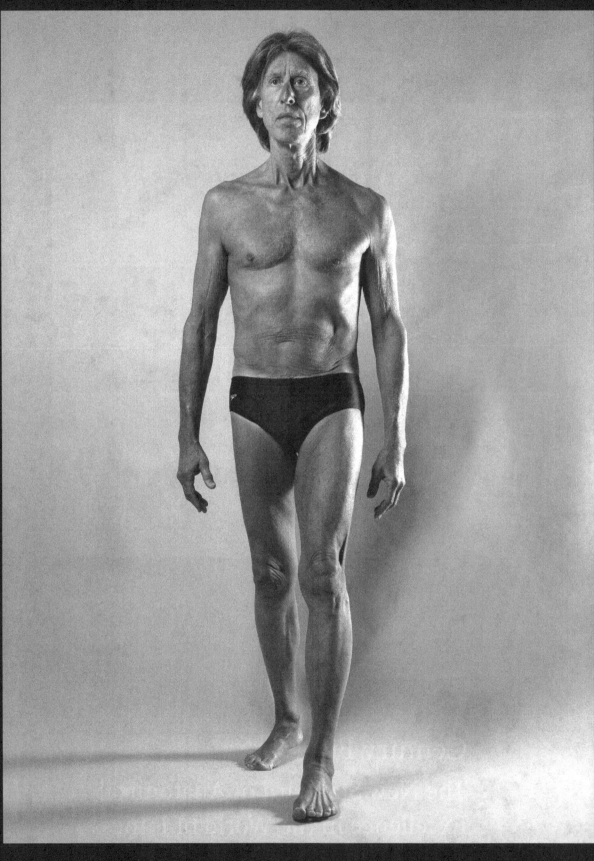

Larry is the first man to achieve and maintain all 8 Essentials of Youth at 75.

8 Essentials of Youth.

1 posture
2 proportion
3 strength
4 nutrition
5 energy
6 agility and flexibility
7 muscle tone
8 cardiovascular capability

"Very few physical culturists practice up to 60 years or more what they preach ... and very few of them can substantiate their claims as reflected in the condition of their bodies"

Joseph Pilates
(1934)

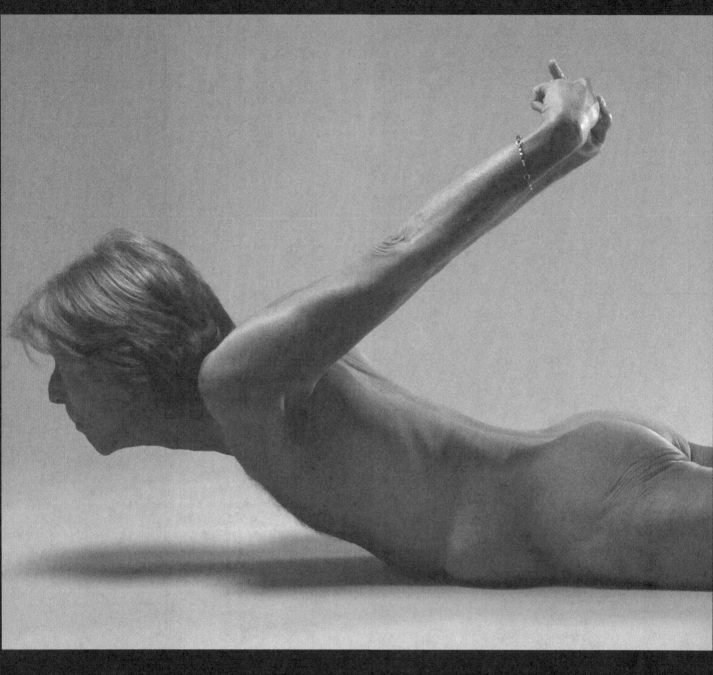

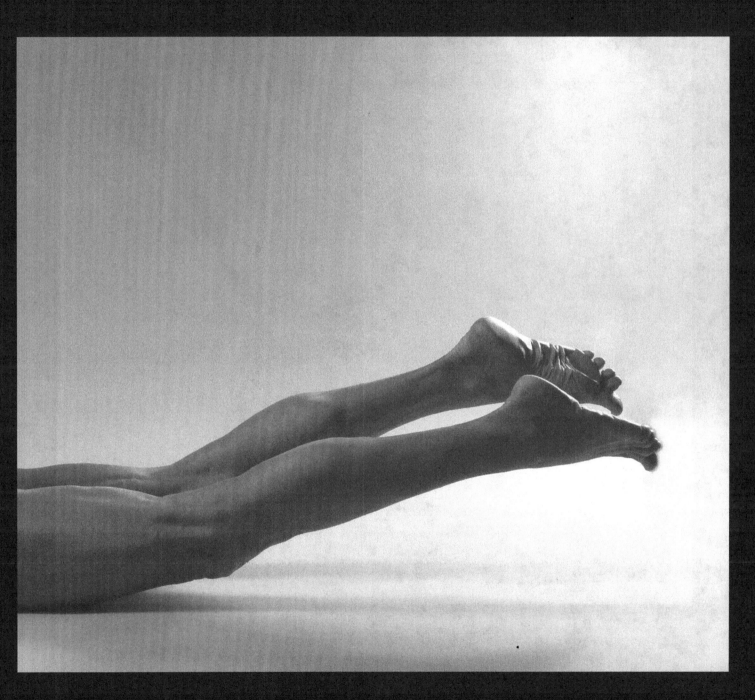

"When it comes to anti-aging, if you can't show it you don't know it"
Larry Nachman
(2013)

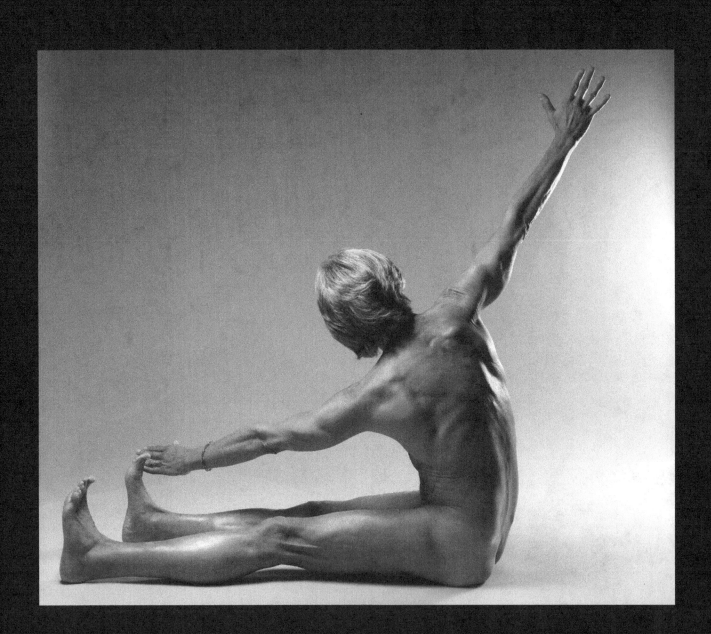

Beyond Yoga · Beyond Pilates

21st Century Fitness is defined by its goal: to reverse the aging process and provide long-lasting youth or a return to youth.

21st Century Fitness is a complete and specific formula of exercise and nutrition. It fills in every piece of the anti-aging puzzle. The exercise portion of the program is designed to systematically stretch and strengthen every muscle group of the body, especially the undermuscles that support the larger muscles.

21st Century Fitness has the resistance and repetition combined with stretch that yoga lacks.

All of this, offering a faster and more efficient road map to success. A standard of excellence that is new to the world of fitness.

75 Should look like this.

Larry Nachman is the first man to achieve and maintain all **8 Essentials of Youth at 75**. He sets the new standard of anatomical and physiological excellence in the world of fitness. Larry represents anti-aging at its best and his 21st Century Fitness formula provides the long-awaited solution to the Fountain of Youth.

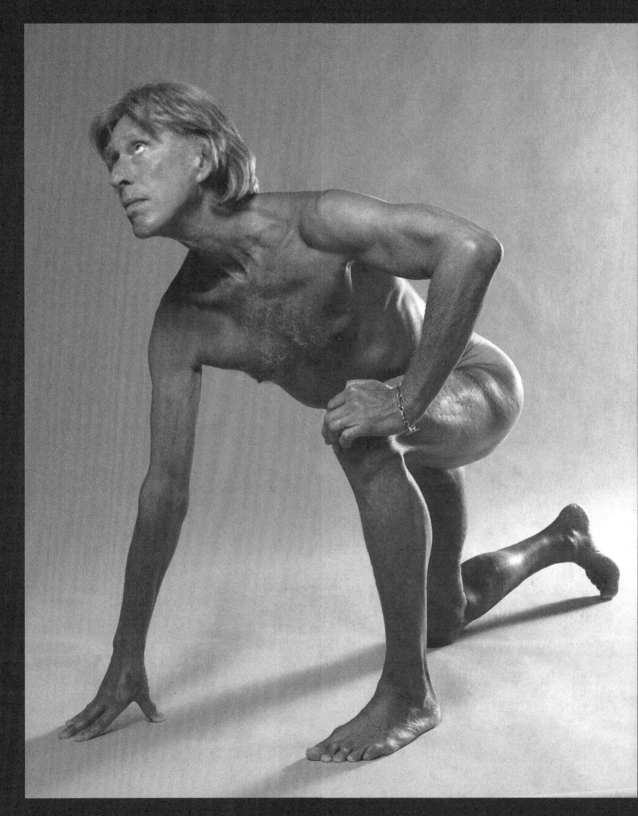

We accept premature aging as the norm rather then the exception.
It is exactly the opposite! Premature aging should be the exception
and viewed by the enlightened as a serious malady.

A different kind of 75.

If your goal is
anti-aging
at its best, and you want to stay
young or return to youth, its
common sense that the only
way to get optimum results is to
ask the man who did it.

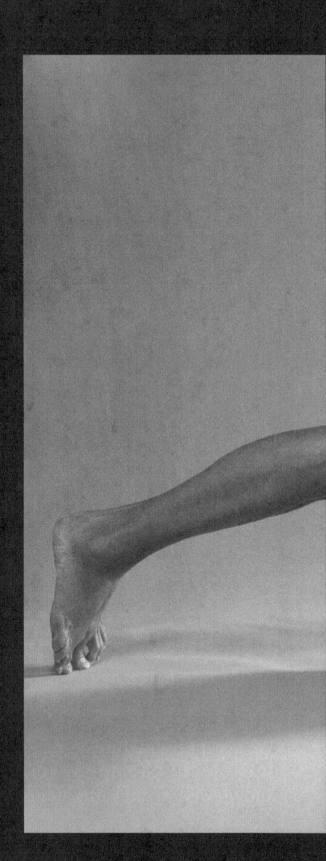

"If your spine is stiff at 25 you are old. If your spine is flexible at 60 you are young."

Joseph Pilates

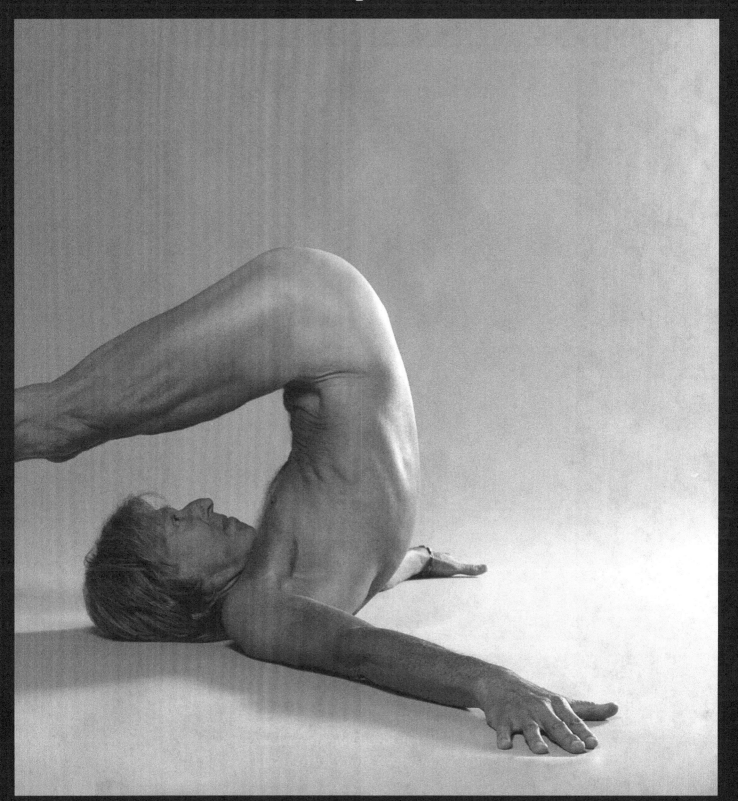

Get this.
Nothing Works Without...

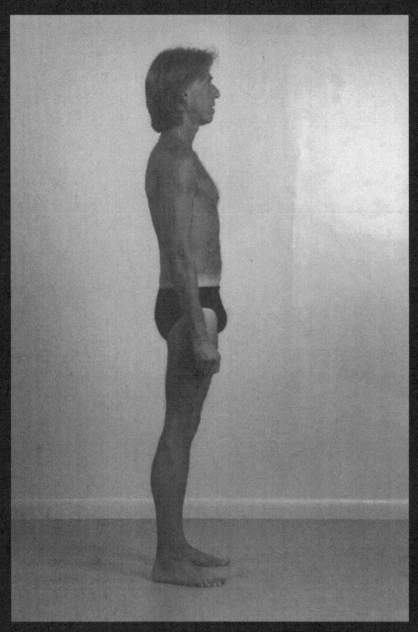

Larry standing tall with straight aligned spine.

BEWARE of middle age spread.....
The side view tells a story unto itself

posture

spine

posture

spine

posture

spine

posture

spine

Its All About
Body Structure **and** Body Frame

The Bullseye of this new direction of
fitness is the structure of the body.
Straight, Tall, Stretched and
Aligned with a Flexible Spine.

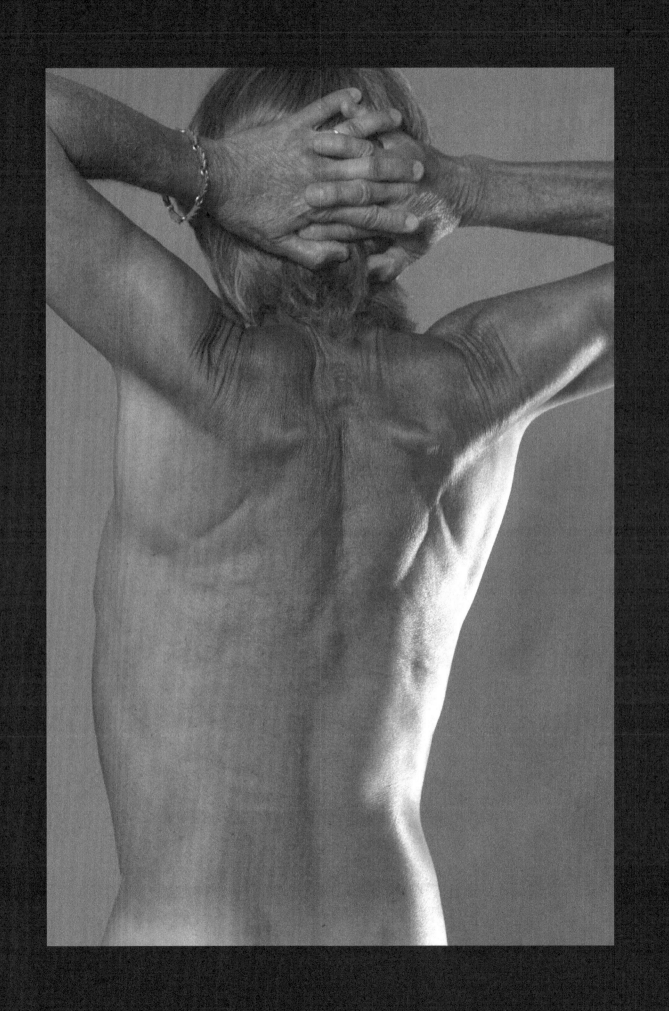

Gravity Defied.
Never before at 75 and over!

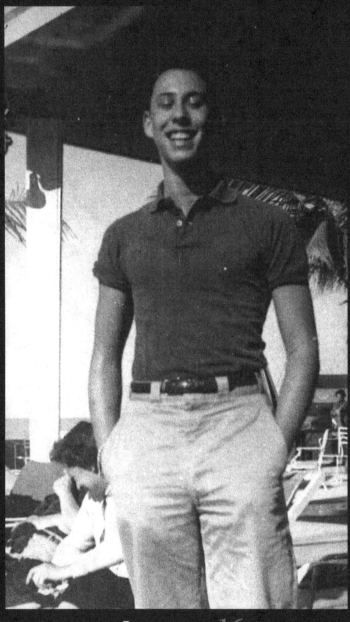

Larry age 16

The ONLY evidenced based formula of exercise and nutrition that offers
sual and living proof that it is possible to defy gravity. Seeing is believi

No longer, Here Today .... Gone Tomorrow

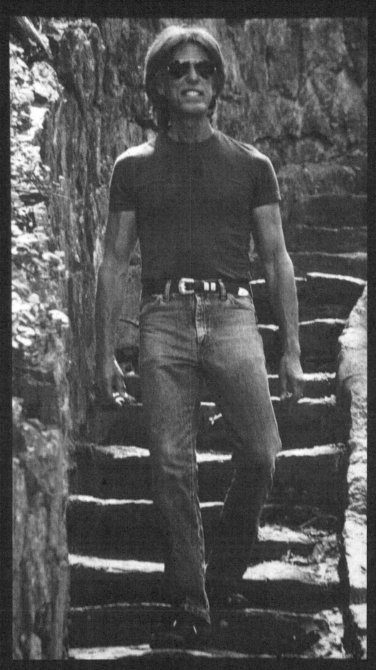

Larry age 75

Will your exercise method allow you to defy gravity?

It is imperative when selecting a method of exercise and nutrition to see proof
that it works. If it worked for Larry, it will work for you!

This is 21st Century Fitness.
Sleek, lean, flexible, agile & toned.

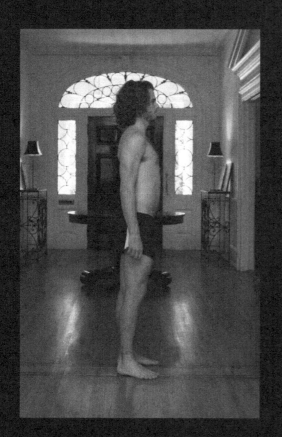 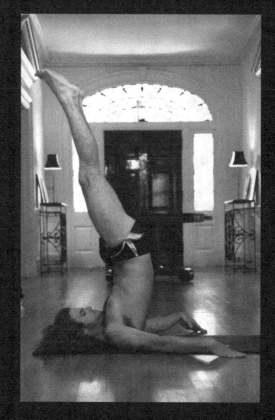

Hagood Granthem age 21

Notice Hagood's square shoulders, high cut chest, slim hips and straight-aligned back. THE NEW BODY: Athletic, long-lean muscle and stretched... Muscle bulk is OUT!

In principle, fitness design is no different than architectural design; both are dictated by function and purpose. In the design of the 21st Century Fitness formula, the purpose is to build an enduring structure — your own body.

"I have been following Larry's 21st Century Fitness program for the last five years. As a high school and college athlete and long-distance runner, I have had a great deal of training. I would describe the training as being the conventional wisdom. Larry's program was an eye opener for me. I had no idea there were so many pieces of the puzzle that were missing from what I had been doing. At the present time , my body is reaching levels beyond my greatest expectations... and his nutrition is outstanding."

Hagood Granthem
(July 2013)

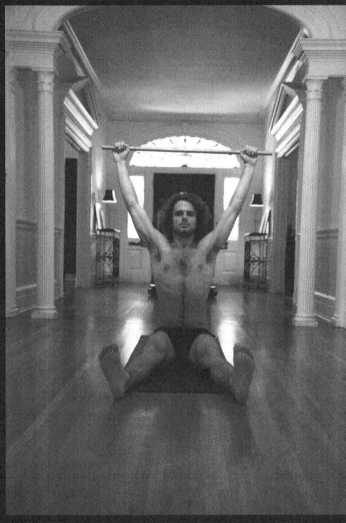

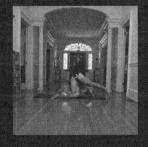 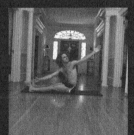

Follow Hagood... He asked the man who did it! Hagood possesses the number 1 essential of youth, which is POSTURE along with the other 7 essentials of youth. If he continues to follow the 21st Century Fitness formula he will have them the rest of his life.

and...This is 21st Century Fitness.

Sleek, lean, flexible, agile & toned.

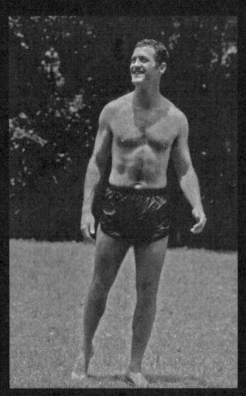

Chuck Jennings
age 36

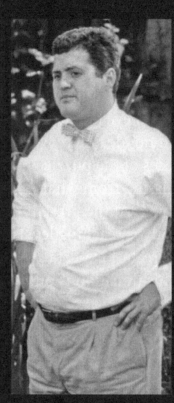

Chuck Jennings
age 35

Notice the change in Chuck's shoulders, chest, hips and back. HIS NEW BODY stands tall and stretched... is lean and athletic. Muscle bulk is OUT!

It is the exactness of the program and the exactness of the movements that makes the 21st Century Fitness FORMULA different from ALL other excerise and nutrition methods.

In the past I had succumbed to that temptation to do more and more, but without success. This time, for some reason, I kept listening to Larry. He told me I didn't need more, that I didn't need anything else, that all I needed was to simply follow the formula. "Do it over and over and over, again and again and again. Don't waiver. You will get the 8 Essentials of Fitness." I did it over and over, again and again. I did not waiver and in twelve months my waist went from a 39 plus to 31 inches. My "genetic" hips and thighs literally melted away. My shoulders grew high, my caved chest became full, and my neck straightened. Physically, I became everything I wanted to be, and it was because of this exact exercise regimen and nutritional plan. Weight loss and a conventional exercise regimen would never have come close to giving me what I have today. It never did.

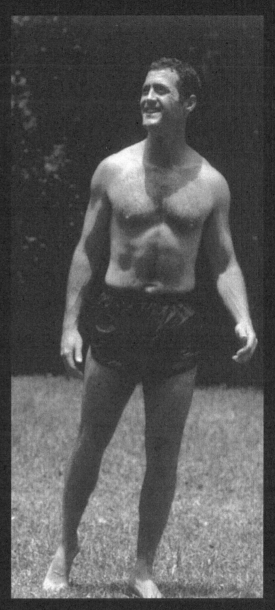

Chuck Jennings

Follow Chuck... He asked the man who did it! Chuck possesses the number 1 essential of youth, which is POSTURE along with the other 7 essentials of youth. If he continues to follow the 21st Century Fitness formula he will have them the rest of his life.

and...This is 21st Century Fitness too.

Sleek, lean, flexible, agile & toned.

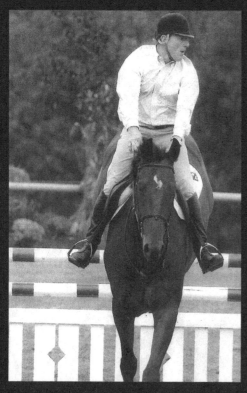

John Boyle
age 67

Eight years-ago, in 2005, I fell off my horse while jumping. My heel was seriously ripped. The doctors did the best they could do under the circumstances, and after physical therapy, I still had a great deal of discomfort. I thought my years of horse back ridding were over. Larry and his 21st Century Fitness formula to the rescue. Two years later, I was perfect. My doctor said he had never seen anyone with my particular injury not limp. In the meantime, my body has totally changed. I have a strong core, lots of flexibility and excellent balance.

The first thing I discovered was the weakness of what Larry termed my "power-house." I thought my stomach muscles were well developed, but Larry showed me how much stronger they could be. As the months progressed I found myself more and more committed to his formula, and I particularly enjoyed seeing the result of using dumbbells.

It is the exactness of the program and the exactness of the movements that makes the 21st Century Fitness FORMULA different from ALL other excerise and nutrition methods.

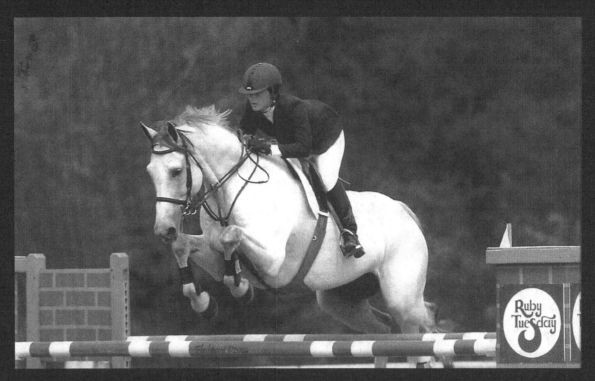

Mary Boyle Steel
age 25

I have been working with Larry over the past 6 years. He knows what other trainers don't, I thought I was getting the best excerise training possible, only to find I was wrong.

My strong an stretched core is the foundation for the improved balance and agility, for which I have been looking. My riding skills have improved dramatically.

Follow John and Mary... They asked the man who did it! John and Mary possess the number 1 essential of youth, which is POSTURE along with the other 7 essentials of youth. If they continue to follow the 21st Century Fitness formula they will have them the rest of their lives.

Follow Me.

and follow the people who asked the man who did it.

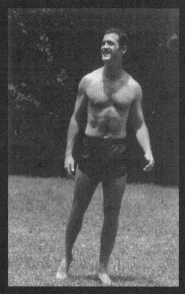

Chuck

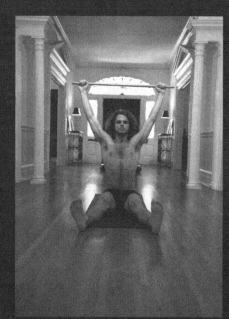

Hagood

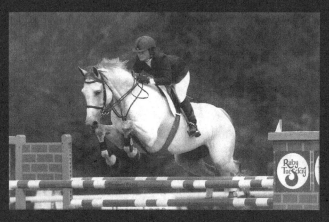

Mary

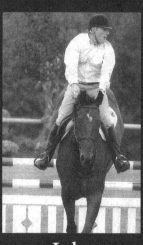

John

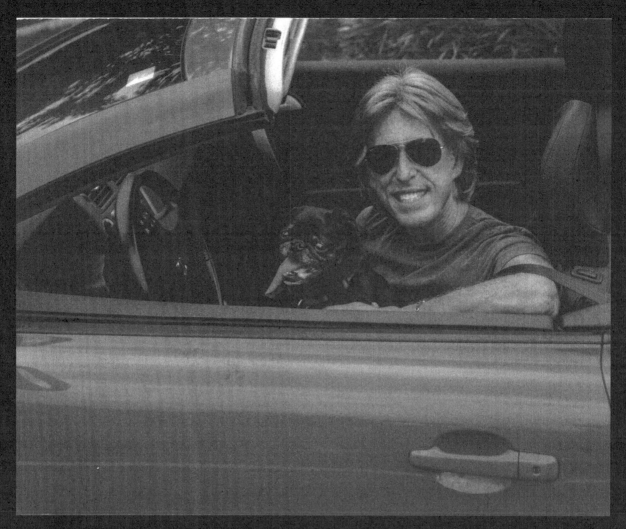

"If you do what I've done, you will get what I've got"

For a lifetime...

I will be your guide to getting younger as you
grow older

Beyond the traditional fitness methods developed in the last century there lies a new dimension of fitness. This new dimension is defined by its goal: to reverse the aging process and provide long-lasting youth.

Unlike traditional fitness methods only the 21st Century Fitness formula incorporates the essentials required to stay young or return to youth. The focus is on the "WHOLE" of the body. THINK; body structure (posture), fascia (deep tissue), telomeres (long nerve endings), muscles (long lean), antioxidants (high levels) It is the "EXACTNESS" of the 21st Century Fitness formula that allows all of the above to work.

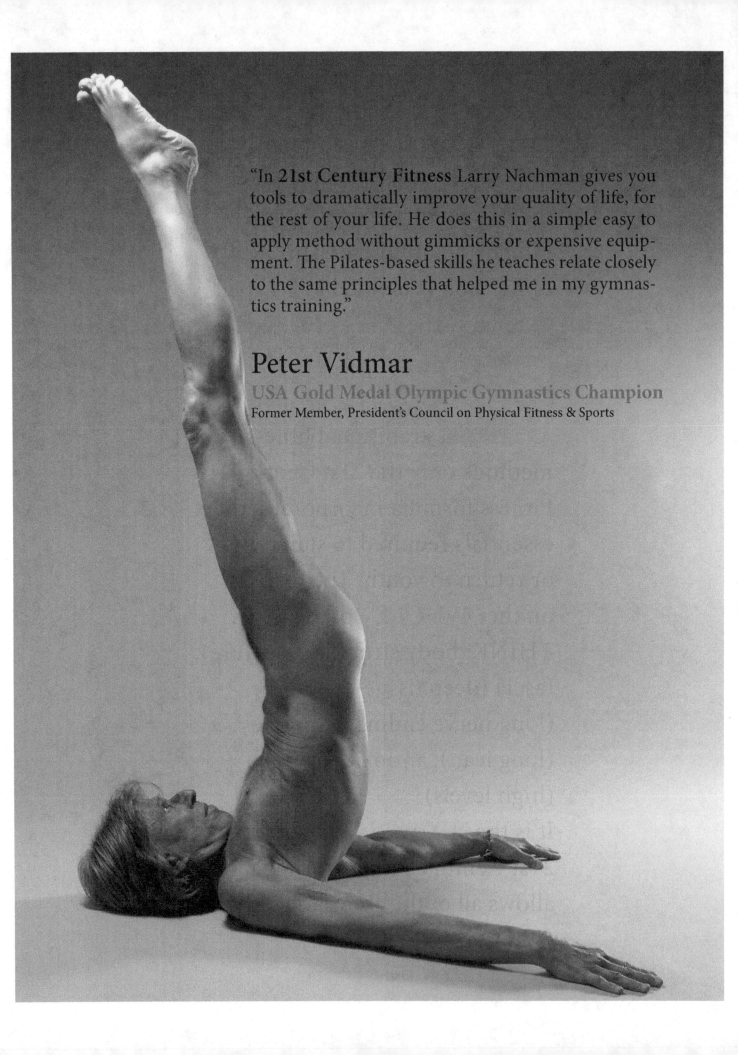

"In **21st Century Fitness** Larry Nachman gives you tools to dramatically improve your quality of life, for the rest of your life. He does this in a simple easy to apply method without gimmicks or expensive equipment. The Pilates-based skills he teaches relate closely to the same principles that helped me in my gymnastics training."

Peter Vidmar
USA Gold Medal Olympic Gymnastics Champion
Former Member, President's Council on Physical Fitness & Sports

Anti - Aging at its best

Right now you are holding in your hands a unique and proven formula for long lasting youth. In front of your eyes you will see Larry Nachman at age 75 and his students who have followed the **21st Century Fitness** formula. They are living proof that it works.

21st Century Fitness provides an answer to a question that has been asked repeatedly through the ages: How can one enjoy youth in his or her later years...even at age 75 and over? This book is a complete formula, a road map to success. It contains every detail on exercise and nutrition required to retain or regain one's youth.

The **21st Century Fitness** formula incorporates the best of 20th century methods, but goes beyond to fill in the missing links. It is a methodology designed to cancel the hit and miss approaches to fitness perpetuated by 20th century conventional wisdom, a school of thought that has led to mass confusion and caused a catastrophe: a senior population physically old long before their time.

This book is designed to develop a new way of thinking about and a new understanding of fitness. My aim is to inspire you to take responsibility for your own body, and for you to come away with a tangible vision of the new dimension of fitness. The "bull'seye" of this new dimension is the **structure of the body:** straight, tall, stretched and aligned with a flexible spine. It is the shift of emphasis from pumped up muscles and bulk to posture and alignment along with sleek, stretched, flexible muscles that breaks the cycle of stagnant thinking and renders most of today's fitness programs ineffective and obsolete.

With **21st Century Fitness** you can join Larry and his students and become part the new young at 75 and over. The formula is fast, effective and can be done anywhere. It's even fun. Read on!

Fit as a Fit 30 Year Old

In 1996, at age 58, Larry debunked the myth that peak physical fitness is only for the young. And he did it in front of 1000 people.

Larry had been invited to enter the American Models and Talent Swimsuit Contest in Hilton Head, South Carolina, but given his age, He harbored more than a few doubts about his chances. At the urging of the woman in charge of the contest, He gave it a shot. Out of the 70 men who were selected to enter, he was the only one over the age of 30. The judges were an international panel made up of heads of leading modeling agencies from New York, Los Angeles, London, Paris, Milan, and Tokyo.

Larry finished in the top ten. The other finalists were all in their 20's. His success in Hilton Head confirmed beyond all doubt the very real value of the **21st Century Fitness** formula, and in fact it was the catalyst for writing this book.

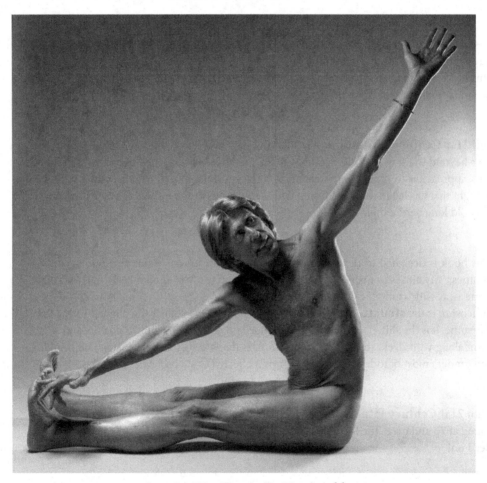

Larry at 75 ... Fit as a Fit 30 year-old

"If you are going to spend the time and energy to exercise, you might as well obtain all 8 Essentials of Youth."

Age vs. Condition

Youth is a condition, not a chronological age. Most people begin to display the signs of aging as early as their teens, yet there are some who seem to get physically younger as they grow chronologically older. It is a paradox that age has nothing to do with physical condition, but that as one grows in wisdom, so can one grow in physical fitness. Imagine a large population of those 75 and over as fit as fit 30 year olds.

21st Century Fitness is for all ages and having all 8 Essentials of Fitness in your 60's and 70's is no longer theory but reality.

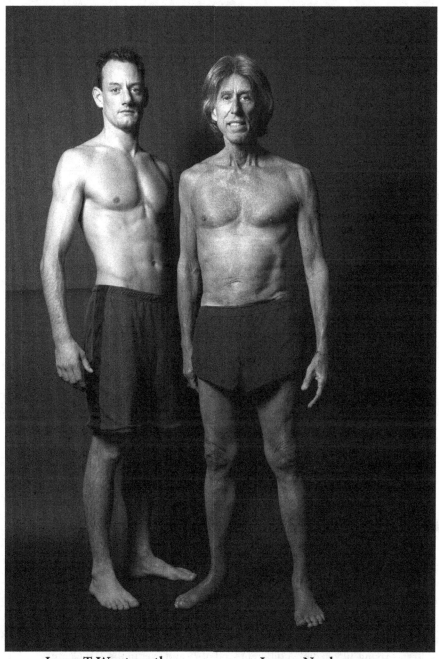

Jason T Wentworth
Age 32

Larry Nachman
Age 75

Young 'til You Die ... 21st Century

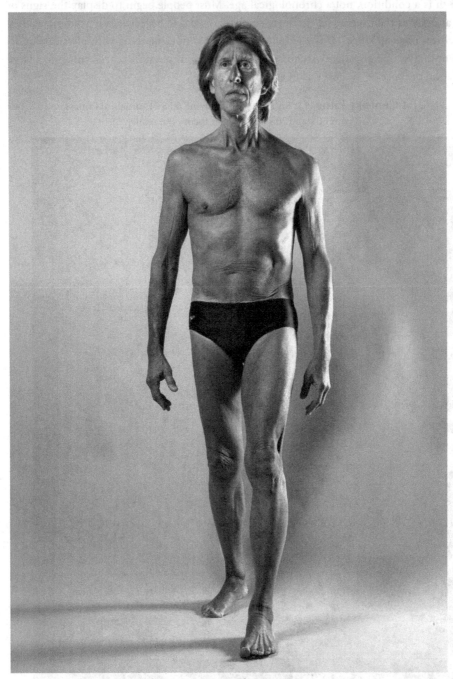

Larry Nachman
21st Century Fitness
Age 75
2013

The goal of "fitness" and the goal of "integrated medicine" has changed. The new thinking
is to stay young 'til you die. A different kind of 75 and over in the 21st Century.

Young 'til You Die ... 20th Century

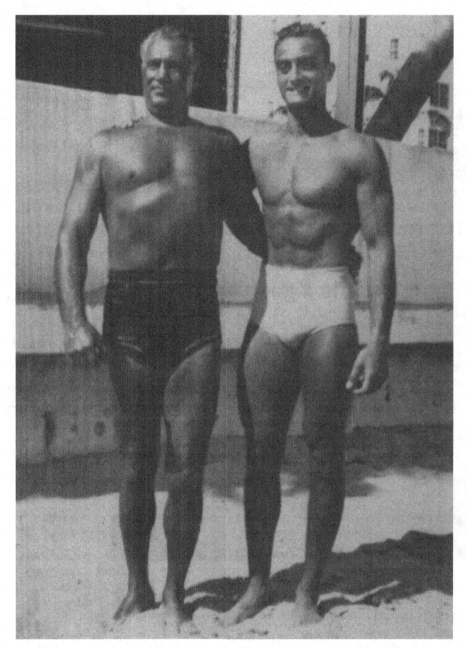

Charles Atlas
(on left)
20th Century Fitness
Age 64
1950

In his younger years, Charles Atlas, held the title as The World's Most Perfect Body. The comparison of Larry and Charles Atlas makes clear the new direction of the 21st Century.

It's Never Too Late. It's Never Too Soon. 21st Century Fitness
For All Ages

Ballet Students Ages 14

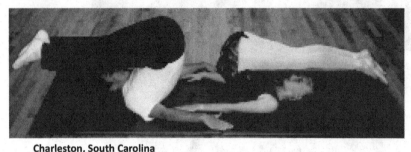

"The ultimate foundation of fitness for all children, and it's fun."

Charleston, South Carolina

Marlene Sher Age 70

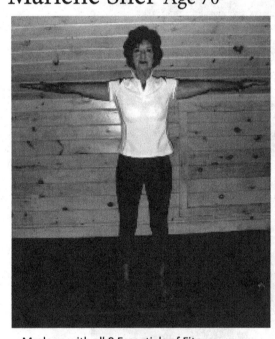

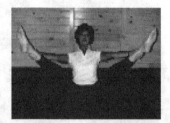

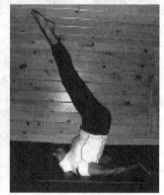

"At age 68 I was heading downhill fast. My energy, flexibility, and strength were fading and I especially noticed problems with my horse-back riding. Thanks to Larry's **21st Century Fitness** formula, I'm as good as new! And as Larry says, I have all 8 Essentials of Youth."

Marlene with all 8 Essentials of Fitness
Columbus, North Carolina

Richard Dowell Age 71

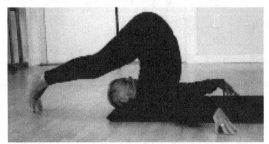

"Starting the **21st Century Fitness** formula at age 68, I had a multitude of physical problems. At age 71, I returned to West Point for my 50th reunion with all 8 Essentials of Youth. I never would have believed it possible."

Richard with all 8 Essentials of Fitness
Charleston, South Carolina

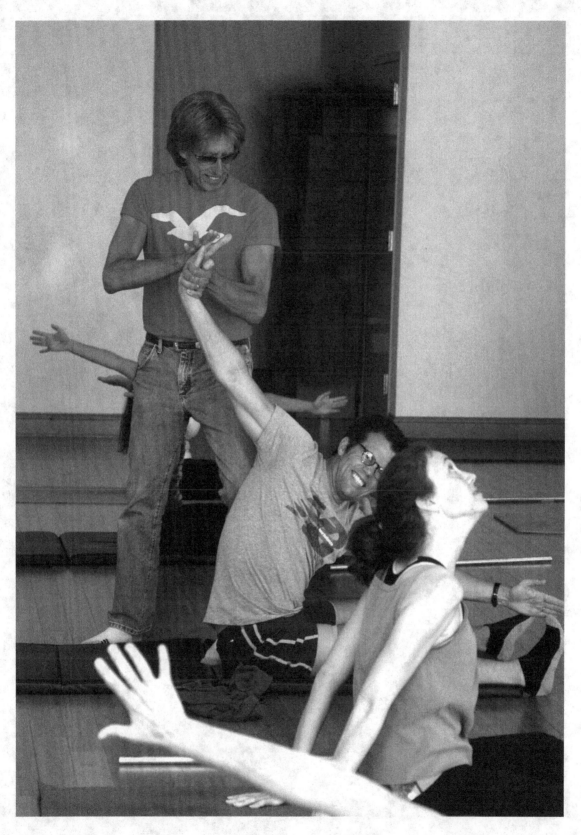

Larry at 75, training students in Charleston, South Carolina

21st Century Fitness is an anti-aging FORMULA, not just another workout or random diet. It is a complete road map for staying young or returning to youth. It is like a recipe .... if something is left out it does not work. It is a new kind of fitness .... much more than a traditional fitness program.

Having ALL 8 Essentials of Youth at 75 and over, or at any age, requires exacting and specific components. Most workouts and diets have chunks of the anti-aging puzzle missing, making it impossible to acquire ALL 8 Essentials of Youth.

There are so many methods one can embrace. Some good .... some bad. Among the good are Yoga/Hot Yoga, treadmill/elliptical, selective weight training/circuit training, Pilates (properly taught, most not), swimming and etc. All good .... BUT NOT GOOD ENOUGH!

WHY?

Not enough core strength.

Not enough specific stretches with resistance and repetition necessary to build the elongated/ strong muscles needed to DEFY GRAVITY over time.

Not enough of the right movements that go deep into the facia (tissue) that promote anti-aging.

NONE of these workouts are enough to provenly allow one to stand tall/ straight and DEFY GRAVITY in their later years, as Larry exhibits (ages 16 and 75).

The wreckage of getting older, in spite of so many fitness and nutrition programs, has been unavoidable until NOW. The 20th Century has been a disaster relating to anti-aging.

But now, with patience and time, it is possible, as you can see with Larry, to get younger as you grow older. It is possible to stay young til you die ..... it is possible to be part of the AGING SOLUTION.

Order this book online at www.trafford.com
or email orders@trafford.com

Most Trafford titles are also available at major online book retailers.

© Copyright 2009, 2015 Larry Nachman.
All rights reserved. No part of this publication may be reproduced, stored in a retrieval system, or transmitted, in any form or by
any means, electronic, mechanical, photocopying, recording, or otherwise, without the written prior permission of the author.

Print information available on the last page.

ISBN: 9781553951339 (sc)
ISBN: 9781426926280 (e)

Because of the dynamic nature of the Internet, any web addresses or links contained in this book may have changed
since publication and may no longer be valid. The views expressed in this work are solely those of the author and do not
necessarily reflect the views of the publisher, and the publisher hereby disclaims any responsibility for them.

Any people depicted in stock imagery provided by Getty Images are models, and
such images are being used for illustrative purposes only.
Certain stock imagery © Getty Images.

Trafford rev. 04/25/2018

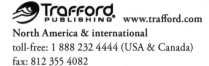 www.trafford.com

North America & international
toll-free: 1 888 232 4444 (USA & Canada)
fax: 812 355 4082

CONTENTS

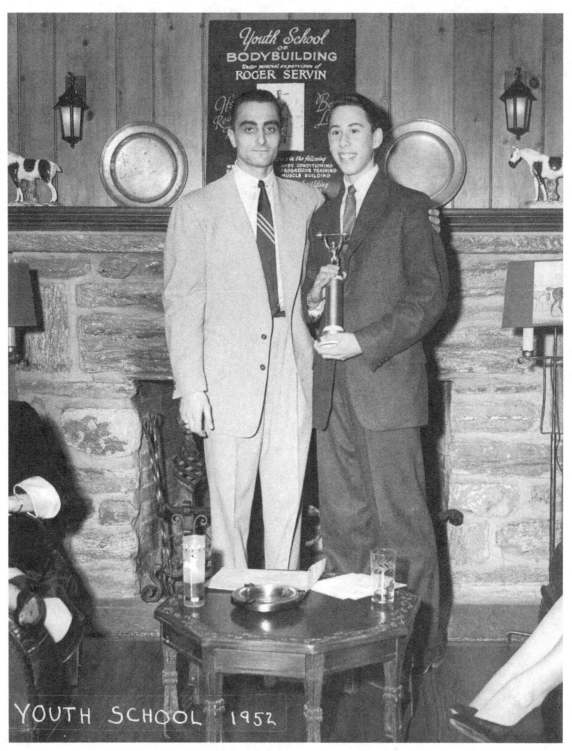

Larry and Roger 1952

A Lifetime in Pursuit of *21st Century Fitness*

I was born in 1937, only a few years after Muscle Beach in Venice, California had become the focal point of fitness in the United States. Those were the days when big muscles and "the Tarzan look" were quite the rage. However, even though weight training was gaining in popularity, in many ways it was still considered avant-garde. Fifteen years later the dust had settled, and weight training was not only accepted, but also adopted as the chief training method in nearly every gym in the country. Despite this national surge of interest, weight training for teenagers remained, if not avant-garde, certainly unusual.

I was one of the rare ones. In 1951, at age 13, I started pumping iron at the Youth School of Bodybuilding in Jenkintown, Pennsylvania, a suburb of Philadelphia. There, under the watchful eye of the young owner/trainer, Roger Servin, I developed my love for fitness. Roger was a bodybuilder and heavily involved in the muscle world, a subculture that was continuing to gain momentum and acceptance. Philadelphia was also home to George Eiferman, who in 1948 earned the title of Mr. America. Soon after, he became Mr. Universe. Although George was certainly an inspiration, it was Roger who was my most important influence. At age 14 I was awarded a handsome trophy that read, "Mr. Youth School, 1952". It was my reward for two years of work to add bulk, shape and definition to my swimmer's body, and it symbolized my dedication to weight training and the emerging body-building scene.

Stretch and Resistance

During this time I was also spending two months every year at summer camp. I had started at age 7, and by the time I was 14 I was the best swimmer there. Because I both swam and lifted weights, I discovered the principle of stretch and resistance. The weight trainers I admired also employed this principle, but where my method for stretch was swimming, theirs was gymnastics and tumbling. This two-tiered principle became an important aspect of the thinking that led me, much later, to make the additions to the Pilates mat, weight resistance, and walking.

As gyms opened across the country the pairing between stretching and resistance was somehow lost. Focus shifted to muscle building and aerobics; overlooked were the connected stretch movements such as gymnastics and swimming. In fact the new gyms rarely made these exercises available. I, too, would succumb to the chrome and glitter of the latest gyms. As a student at Tulane University in New Orleans, I joined just such a facility, the first of many to which I would eventually belong.

In 1960 I moved to New York City, and shortly upon arrival I made my first visit to the Pilates Studio on 8th Avenue in Hell's Kitchen. Joseph Pilates was alive at the time - very much alive - and he was working with a client at one end of the room. Pilates' wife Clara, dressed in a starched nurse's uniform, greeted me with a heavy German accent. Everything about this studio seemed strange; there were weird machines that looked like they may have been used in the Spanish Inquisition. Clara gave me a quick rundown on the Pilates philosophy and asked me if I would like to make an appointment for a workout. I said, "Not right now. I'll call you." Of course I didn't. I was cocky about my fitness knowledge and rejected Pilates to return to my comfortable, traditional training at a more conventional gym.

For the rest of my 20s and into my 30s I worked out diligently at a variety of gyms. It is important to understand that at this time I was not a "hothouse flower." I lived it up and partied with the best of 'em. I loved my down-home Carolina cooking: lots of fried chicken, macaroni and cheese, ham biscuits, etc. In spite of all of this I looked good, but at age 35 things started to happen.

The Crossover Age

To my amazement and frustration, no matter what I did or how hard I worked out, my posture and flexibility were going. I was "thickening" and "dropping". My knees ached. I couldn't turn my head properly. I didn't look or perform at all as I had in my youth. Contributing to my decline were results from two stomach operations I underwent at age 30. In both cases the 12 inch incisions through the abdominal muscles caused my doctors to offer opinions that my stomach would never again be flat. To counter this I added more to my weight resistance, swimming and jogging routines. I tried bicycling, Judo, Yoga, and Aerobics. You name it, and I tried it. Even my old reliance on stretch and resistance, swimming and weights, was not enough. None of these worked to stop the decline I was experiencing. I was under the preconceived notion that all I had to do was increase my workout schedule, but that only resulted in making things worse. My time was being eaten up. And as I realize now, I was working hard to stay unfit.

Return to Pilates

Around this time I remembered my short visit to the Pilates Studio more than a decade before. I remembered, too, the words of Clara Pilates: "STRETCHED...TALL...FLEXIBLE...ALIGNED" and "EVERYTHING CENTERS ON THE SPINE." So in 1973, I returned to the studio, at age 36, that was then under the direction of Romana Kryzanowska, who had been handed the reigns by Joseph Pilates himself. To this day it is Romana's standards that set her a world apart from most certified Pilates instructors. And to have studied under her for so long was a privilege. Within a few months I was getting exactly what I wanted — and what I needed! My body was reawakening to its former youthfulness, and over time I felt my agility and flexibility return. I was standing taller, and not only did I start to feel years younger, I looked it!

But training at Pilates was work! I would have pools of perspiration surrounding me after a non-stop hour of their specialized workout routines. THE REFORMER...THE MAT...and then the trainer would say, "TO THE TOWER...TO THE BARREL." Finally, just as I thought I had reached the end, I would hear, "TO THE CADILLAC!". I would feel like crawling to the shower. Eventually I had THE REFORMER, THE CADILLAC, LITTLE BARREL, and BIG BARREL built for my new home in Greenville, South Carolina because I was commuting between there and New York. As you can see, Pilates had become an important part of my life!

It was now clearly evident that at age 35 I had reached what I referred to earlier as the crossover age. Up until this point most exercise regimens will yield partial and sometimes nearly complete fitness. Past 35, however, the body's changes are insidious, and to maintain or attain the essentials of youth in one's later years one needs a program of specific design. That is exactly what I received training under Romana. Not only did I return to the youthfulness I had enjoyed in my 20s, but I became more flexible and more agile as I climbed plane after plane of sustained, life-long fitness.

The *21st Century Fitness* Formula

At age 47 I realized my lifestyle was preventing me from performing the traditional Pilates workout routine. My demanding business schedule, which included a considerable amount of travel, was the chief culprit. I needed a program that offered me fast, efficient workouts that could be done anywhere, at any time, with no equipment requirements. To make the needed changes I put my years of experience to work. It required a new way to think about fitness. I tested, edited and rejected, stripping away the excess. The adage held true: less was more, and as I refined this efficient new formula it became apparent that what was not in it was as important as what was in it.

It is important to note that within a few years of developing this new formula I suffered another fitness decline due to an illness. I became borderline emaciated and lost a good bit of muscle tone. My body had aged prematurely. At this point the *21st Century Fitness* formula was put to the critical test. Having recovered from my illness, I began working out again. With patience and time the formula worked, and I was able to achieve the level of fitness I had enjoyed at the Pilates Studio and carry forth those results even today.

21st Century Fitness

The new attitude about aging.
The new way to think about fitness.

The time has come to embrace the new understanding that modern fitness, **21st Century Fitness**, is evidence-based and the standard of excellence is having all *8 Essentials of Fitness* at age 75 and over.

The time has come to understand the new thinking —

Seeing Is Believing ...
Visual Proof ...
Reality vs. Theory.

The new battle cry — follow the winner.
I continually tell my students, ***"if you do what I have done you will get what I got."*** So many have accomplished the goal of **21st Century Fitness**. It took faith, trust, patience, and dedication, but everyone of them will tell you that it has turned their lives around completely. They now believe 75 really is the new young.

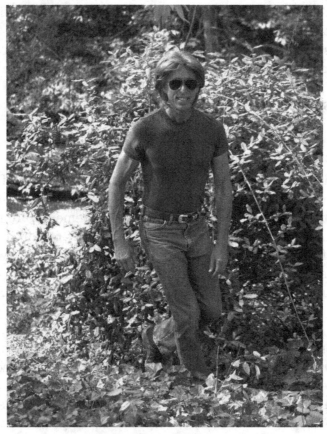

Follow The Winner
"You will get what I got"

21st Century Fitness: Beyond Pilates

In a country obsessed with the illusion of fitness, methods change as quickly as fashion trends. Most people go through the exercise and nutrition maze as they would a salad bar, trying a little of this and a little of that. Rarely, though, do they get what they really want or need — even if they're lucky enough to know what that is.

Elaborate gyms rarely have the answers, and personal trainers are expensive. Also, they are only as good as the training they received. Home exercise equipment is usually only a partial solution. Jogging is hard on the joints. It can be frustrating and down right confusing.

Today a fitness method first introduced in America almost 80 years ago has become the newest craze. But is it a craze?

For decades the Pilates Method has been a secret of the physical elite: choreographers George Balanchine and Martha Graham, movie stars Sharon Stone, Julia Roberts and Melanie Griffith, the San Francisco Forty-Niners and Cincinnati Bengals, and ballet companies in New York, Philadelphia and Atlanta. All have reaped the benefits of Pilates.

I became a student of the Pilates Method in 1973 when only a select few in and around the New York City area had the time and resources to avail themselves to what has since been labeled a fitness breakthrough. I found it to be everything I sought in a fitness regimen, and I had been devoted to a life of fitness since the age of 13. The Pilates Method took me to levels I never imagined possible, but I realized that in order to maintain these levels it would require more time than I could allow due to demands of work and family. How could I reconcile the seemingly conflicting demands of fitness and life?

I began to experiment. From the universe of fitness regimens, I tested, edited, rejected and refined. In the end, I produced a formula that offers fast, efficient workouts that can be done anywhere, at any time, with no equipment requirements. Better yet, these workouts can be accomplished in an average of 30 minutes a day. I called my new formula *21st Century Fitness* because, while it incorporates the best of 20th century methods, it goes beyond to fill in the gaps that have long been missing.

> **Beyond the traditional methods developed over the last one hundred years lies a new dimension of fitness. This new dimension is defined by its goal: To reverse the aging process and provide long-lasting youth.**

What is *21st Century Fitness*?

21st Century Fitness is a method that will provide you with all *8 Essentials of Fitness* into your later years.

As early as 1945 Joseph Pilates was championing a realistic concept of long-lasting youth. In that year he gave a copy of his book, **Return To Life Through "Contrology,"** to one of his students, Jeannie Cerni. The book is inscribed, *"To Jeannie - Everlasting youth to you and yours through 'Contrology'".* The essence of Pilates' teaching is to extend youth far beyond the normally accepted limits. After almost half a century, Jeannie Cerni, now a student of mine, is adept at the exercises of *21st Century Fitness*. She has the posture, coordination, energy, agility and flexibility that enable her, at age 81, to remain an accomplished ballroom dancer.

Inscription to Jeannie Cerni
From Joseph Pilates, 1945

Today, Joseph Pilates' message of long-lasting youth is especially relevant because people are living longer. Instead of living robust, active lives, however, many will spend their later years as medical dependents. They will merely endure a life of second-class citizenship in our youth-oriented society. There is a choice: the fitness of youth or the premature frailty of the aged.

Most people do age prematurely because they believe that traditional fitness methods actually work. In most cases though, they don't. If they did, we would see a large population of those 60 and older who have the eight essentials of fitness. What we see is the opposite. Without a program that includes specific exercises and nutrition proven to obtain these eight essentials, it is very unlikely people will discover them on their own. What's needed is a program, *a specific formula* to become *8 Essential Fit*, which is exactly what *21st Century Fitness* offers. The solution lies in three words: *proven, specific and formula.*

A WORD OF CAUTION: fitness is an elusive concept because so many are deceived by the facade of fitness. For example, the ten-mile-a-day jogger, full of stamina and energy, might have slumping shoulders and very little flexibility. A person may play a good game of tennis, but, with a 40 inch waist and large hips, he or she will fail the test of proportion. The body-builder might have large muscles, but what about agility and flexibility?

6

So you see, while these people may possess some pieces to the fitness puzzle, they lack the others. As you progress through the **21st Century Fitness** formula, you will recognize the following components as being essential in obtaining the goal of long-lasting youth.

The 8 Essentials of 21st Century Fitness

Posture: alignment and straightness of the spine

Cardio-Vascular Capability: sustained ability of the heart and blood vessels to carry oxygen to the blood cells

Energy: inherent power, a capacity of action; in physics energy is defined as the capability of doing work

Agility & Flexibility: grace and quickness; muscle elasticity; the ability to use muscles and joints through the full range of movement; a flexible spine

Muscle Tone: how much is lean mass? How much is fat?

Proportion: 8" to 10" waist to chest spread on men; 4" to 5" bust to waist to hips spread on women

Strength: muscle fitness; the force muscle or muscles can produce in one contraction; power, the amount of work done in a given period of time

Nutrition: nourishment to maximize digestion and energy; to maintain and regenerate blood cells; works with exercise to create healthy metabolism

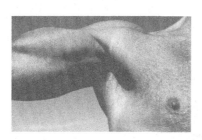 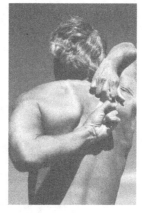

Sleek vs. Bulky: Elongated muscles provide for agility, flexibility and suppleness. The floor work of *21st Century Fitness* provides the foundation for attaining a long, lean, stretched-out, "open" body — the earmarks of long lasting youth.

Fitness: It is like buying a diamond

When buying a diamond, we do not simply walk into a jewelry store and say, "I'll take that one."

The knowledgeable buyer knows that diamonds are available in a wide variety of qualities, defined by specific standards. The same is true of fitness. The qualities of fitness are defined by specific standards.

Most people do not think of fitness in this way. Most people think of fitness in vague terms. They embark on programs without having clarity of vision and do not understand that fitness, like a diamond, is defined by specifics.

In most fitness programs, people are given exact instructions on what to do, but are not given the specifics of the results. They are told they will get "fit." But what does that mean? What fit? Cardio-fit? Muscular fit? Flexibility fit? To what specific standards? When? Will they be *8 Essential Fit* at age 75 and over? Are they paying the price of a fine diamond to get a flawed stone?

21st Century Fitness specifically defines the eight essentials of fitness. Not only does *21st Century Fitness* define the *8 Essentials*, it offers a specific formula to achieve specific results in 30 minutes a day.

As with the standards for a fine diamond, the *21st Century Fitness* formula offers standards for fitness as demonstrated by Larry Nachman at age 75.

The Standard:
ALL 8 ESSENTIALS OF FITNESS

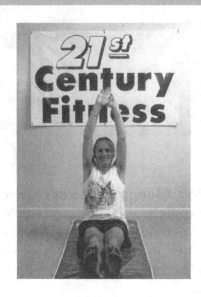

21st Century Fitness: A New Methodology

Through the ages, as men and women have sought ideal fitness, the experts have been in constant debate over the best methods to achieve strength, endurance, flexibility and an aesthetically pleasing shape. Eastern methods such as Yoga and Tai Chi emphasize mental relaxation, suppleness and breathing, while Western methods emphasize muscle bulk, strength and endurance. There are die-hard advocates for each. I've found the answer lies in both. *21st Century Fitness* is a hybrid of Eastern and Western methods of exercise, a **balanced** combination of stretch and weight resistance. To these I've added three more elements so that the formula provides every detail required to stay young or to regain youth.

The *21st Century Fitness* formula is a simple program. These elements include an edited version of the original 34 "Contrology" exercises developed by Joseph Pilates (now the Pilates mat), additional exercises of my design (fill-ins), hand weights, walking and nutrition.

The Five Elements of *21st Century Fitness*

Floor work is the foundation. It strengthens and builds control of the center of the body. The abdomen, lower back and buttocks provide stability as the rest of the body moves through a variety of range-of-motion and resistance exercises.

Weight resistance is designed specifically for upper body strength to complement the strength acquired from floor work.

Fill-in exercises provide the crowning touch to what has been accomplished with the floor work and weight resistance.

Walking concentrates on the legs and the cardiovascular system. Additional benefits for the legs and hips.

Nutrition is a vital part of the *21st Century Fitness* formula. Without it, one cannot achieve all *8 Essentials of Fitness,* especially in one's later years.

Principles of the *21st Century Fitness* Formula

Powerhouse Muscles: (the six-pack) the focus is to develop the muscles in the center of the body that connect the abdomen to the lower back and the buttocks.

Long-lasting Youth: all 8 Essentials of Fitness at 75 and over.

Age vs. Condition: youth is a condition, not a chronological age. Some people exhibit the signs of aging as early as their teens, while there are those who seem to get physically younger as they age chronologically. Chronological age has nothing to do with fitness.

Connected vs. Isolated Movements: the only way to achieve a straight, flexible and stretched spine is with exercises that are connected movements from head to toe. This is contrary to conventional, isolated movements such as working arms, legs, or neck separately.

Stretching with Resistance: the objective is for the stretched muscle to hold its stretch. This can only be done when the muscle is stretched with resistance, which is achieved through the force of gravity.

Sleek vs. Bulk: elongated, flexible, stretched muscles as opposed to short, tight, bulky muscles

Economy of Motion: achieving the most effective results in relation to energy expended. There are no superfluous movements in the *21st Century Fitness* formula.

Less is More: to achieve all *8 Essentials of Fitness* with the least number of exercises in the shortest amount of time. Effectiveness is the goal. What is in the formula is as important as what is not.

The Crossover Age: the critical time in person's life at which a specific formula is required to achieve all *8 Essentials of Fitness* and long-lasting youth (age 35).

Appearance vs. Performance: looking good is not the same as being fit. A person may look good, but fail to possess all *8 Essentials*.

Proof: my method works. My students and I are the proof.

Repetition: the success of the *21st Century Fitness* formula lies in repetition. It is a precise formula, and when performed as directed, provides all eight essentials. Nothing more is needed!

Tincture of Time: the *21st Century Fitness* formula will bring immediate positive results, and these results continue to improve with the passage of time. Just like a fine wine, we continue to get better right through our later years.

Criteria for the *21st Century Fitness* Formula

Most people lead busy lives. Finding time for fitness can be a problem. Since time and convenience are important factors to consider, *21st Century Fitness* incorporates five criteria to enable anyone seeking total fitness to use the formula:

Shortness of Time: fast, efficient workouts

Flexibility of Place: workouts that can be done anywhere, any time, even when traveling

Easy to Do: uncomplicated workouts; the only requirement is patience

Minimal Equipment: one pair of dumbbells

No Dues or Fees

This is *21st Century Fitness*

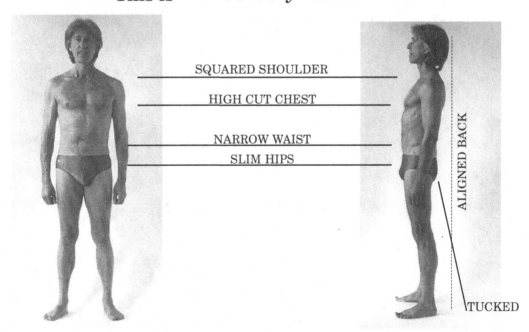

SQUARED SHOULDER

HIGH CUT CHEST

NARROW WAIST

SLIM HIPS

ALIGNED BACK

TUCKED

Larry Nachman at age 75

In principle, fitness design is no different than architectural design; both are dictated by function and purpose. In the design of *21st Century Fitness* formula, the purpose is to build an enduring structure — your own body.

What Fit?

The Goal: *8 Essential Fit* at 75 and over.
The Result: See below center — Larry Nachman *8 Essential Fit* at 75.

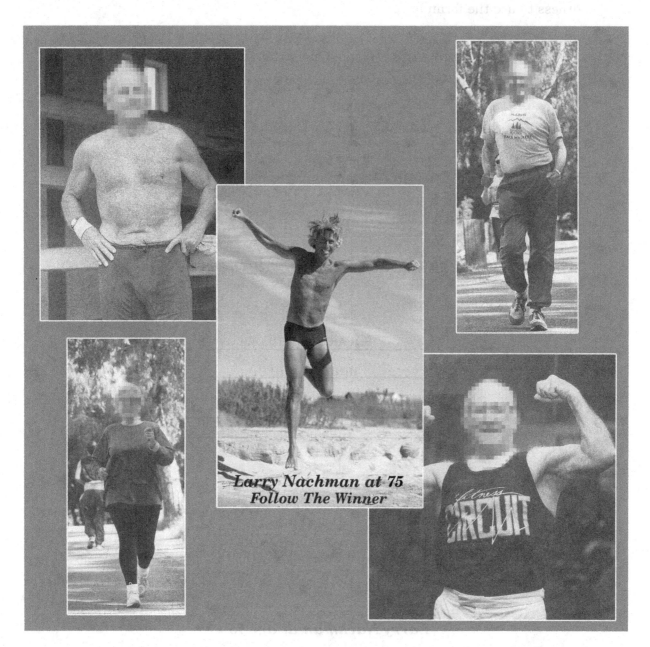

Larry Nachman at 75
Follow The Winner

We Have Choices On How We Look And Move In Our 60's and 70's.
Larry's *21st Century Fitness* allows you to have a different kind of body.
STRETCHED, FLEXIBLE, TONED, STRONG.

DO NOT SETTLE FOR LESS.

Keys to Understanding *21st Century Fitness*

> **Structure/Posture**
> **Isolated vs. Connected**
> **Powerhouse**
> **T-Zone**

As the architect begins his design with the *foundation* and the *structure* of his building, the *21st Century Fitness* formula begins with the *foundation* and the *structure* of the body. The architect's first concern is for the integrity of the structure; the adornments will come later. In the *21st Century Fitness* formula, the integrity of the body design is based on a straight, aligned spine - the *structure* with the foundation to support it so that it *endures*.

Structure/Posture

The single most essential component of long-lasting youth is standing tall, the alignment of the spine resulting from correct posture. The floor work in *21st Century Fitness* is the foundation of good posture. It is the synchronized connected movements coupled with the resistance in floor work that is the key to standing tall.

Isolated vs. Connected

The head-to-toe connected movements of the floor work of the *21st Century Fitness* formula is the only way I know to change the structure and alignment of the body within the criteria of the program (shortness of time, flexibility of place, ease of workout, and minimal equipment).

The vast majority of 20th century fitness programs emphasize *isolated* movements. An isolated movement in fitness is the concentration on one muscle or one group of muscles at a time—-abs, arms or legs—-as opposed to exercising the *whole body* in one continuous movement, as in the floor work. By focusing on *isolated* muscles, these "last century" programs fail to include the most important element of exercise if one wants to change the structure of the body: *connected* movements coupled with *resistance*. The traditional *isolated* stretching movements, which lack the *resistance* factor, do not allow the stretched muscle to hold its position, and thus the body structure does not change. It will bounce back just like a rubber band.

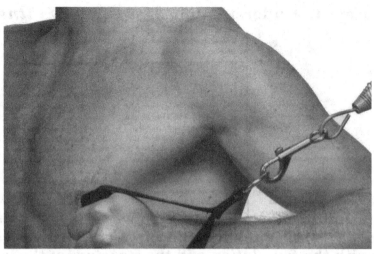

Isolated Exercise
(i.e. arms only, abs only, chest only, legs only)

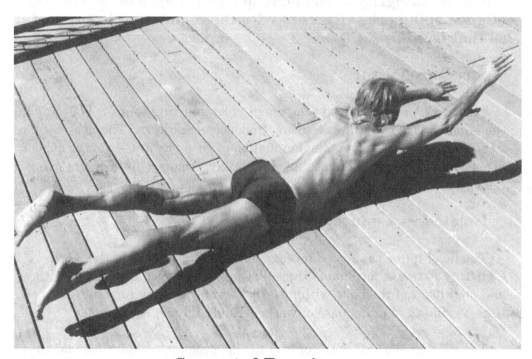

Connected Exercise
<u>*whole*</u> **body movement head to toe**

   The *connected* movements of floor work allow for the re-shaping of the body. This process takes time and patience, but it will happen. Even those who are genetically predisposed to large hips, heavy thighs, and protruding stomachs can eliminate these conditions. I have never seen a so-called "genetic pear" that could not be corrected.

Powerhouse

Core to **21st Century Fitness** is the Powerhouse. Without a strong midsection, the body will not stand tall in its later years. The midsection is between the ribcage and the line across the hips, which also includes the lower back. The most common mistake people make related to "fitness" is asking which exercises are best for the stomach or lower back. **It is the combination of all 21st Century Fitness exercises that leads to a strong stomach and lower back.**

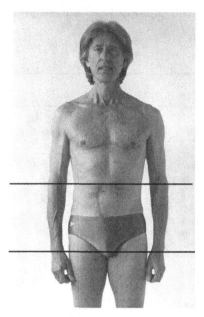

T-Zone

The objective of **21st Century Fitness** in relation to the chest and ribcage is to bypass the traditional loss of definition between the upper abdomen and chest. The goal is to maintain a high chest line and ribcage and a defined upper abdomen. Again, floor work is the only method I know that will give you the permanent stretch to create a strong, defined T-Zone.

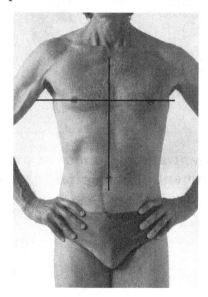

A Different Kind of Body

The *21st Century Fitness* formula changes the focus of fitness from muscles to posture, and it's the floor work that gives you a different kind of body, especially as you get older. This change of emphasis allows for the rebuilding of the body's structure and provides endurance, which is critical to reversing the aging process. Your appearance becomes taller, leaner, straighter, toned, stretched and in proportion. Your performance becomes energetic, stronger, and more flexible with an improved cardiovascular capability. It is this different kind of body that allows you to stay young.

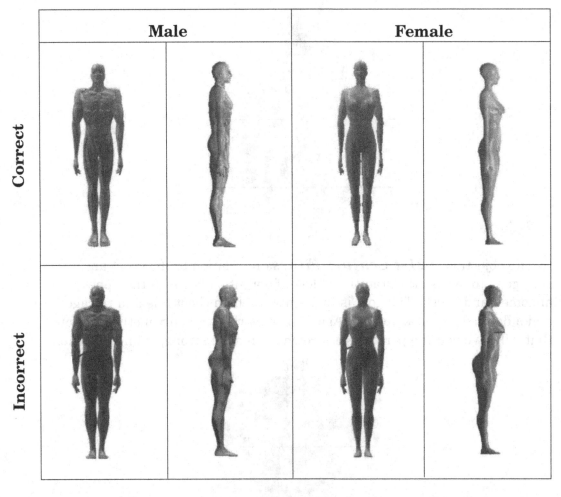

The single most essential component of long-lasting youth is standing tall, an alignment of the spine resulting from correct posture.

Energy Meridians

Meridians are energy points. As we age, meridians become blocked, and this can happen as early as one's 20s. The floor work of *21st Century Fitness* is designed to keep our meridians open and connected, just like well conducted circuits of electricity. The key in doing this is the connected head to toe exercises. It is the attention to not only the external, but also the internal that develops A **Different Kind Of Body** and allows you to be 8 *Essential Fit.*

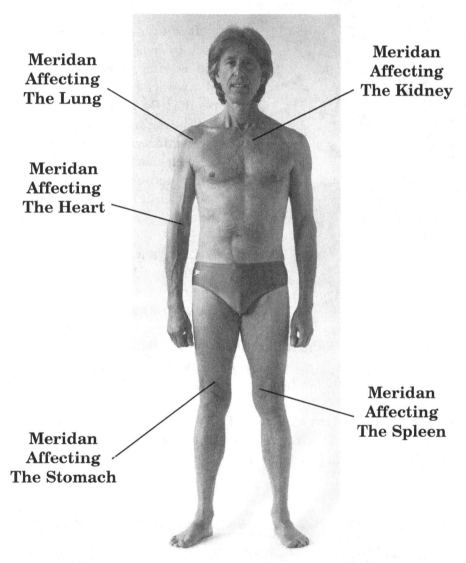

Meridan Affecting The Lung

Meridan Affecting The Kidney

Meridan Affecting The Heart

Meridan Affecting The Spleen

Meridan Affecting The Stomach

"When you slouch, you crowd your organs. But when your body is in alignment, your organ systems have the proper space to function."

Dr. Young C. Yi

ANTI - AGING AT ITS BEST

Join the "Incognito Oldies"

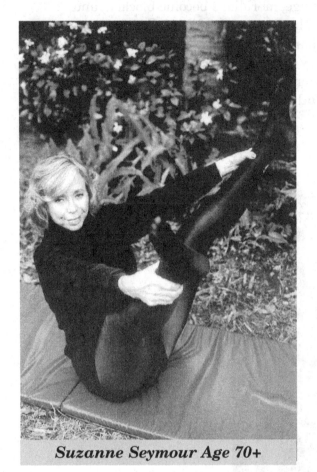

Suzanne Seymour Age 70+

There comes a time in every life when our youthful powers decline. Usually this starts to occur in our mid to late thirties: the crossover age. And, despite the romantic lyrics of poets and songwriters, the crossover age is a time of inner panic for most.

It is a time when many people flock to spas, gyms, trainers and the myriad of cures for aging. Many work hard, but do they get results? Do they end up achieving the *8 Essentials of Fitness* in their later years? Some get "fitter," but most "work hard to stay unfit" and end up with some of the essentials of fitness, but not all eight.

Until now, Pilates as taught by Romana Kryzanowska in the original New York studio, was the only other answer to bypassing the aging process. There are some who have achieved reasonable success with other methods but it usually requires enormous amounts of time and energy. "Real People", those with jobs, families, & social pressures are usually left behind if it takes too much time and energy.

Other than *21st Century Fitness* I know of no other formula of exercise and nutrition that is as effective and efficient where one can achieve all *8 Essentials of Fitness* at 75 and over.

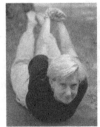 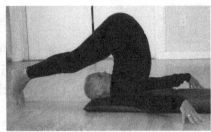 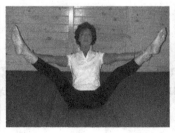 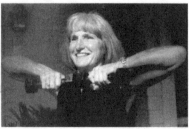

The *21st Century Fitness* Formula

When one thinks of great architectural design—-the Parthenon at Athens, the Pyramids of Egypt and the Yucatan, St. Paul's Cathedral in London, the Chrysler and Empire State buildings in New York—-we are reminded of the genius that built them. These architects understood that *endurance* is the first test of their art.

The Empire State Building was an architectural breakthrough. Its height of 102 stories was considered impossible. The engineering that enabled its construction was so precise, and the synchronization of engineering and construction principles was so intricately woven, that it set a new standard. It was the *precision, balance, and repetition* of one floor a day that resulted in that monument to our country's greatness. It's these same elements—-*precision, balance and repetition*—-in the context of the *21st Century Fitness* formula that provide the eight essentials for another feat of *endurance*, long-lasting youth.

If a building's endurance is the first purpose of architecture, then so is a body's *endurance* is the first purpose of a fitness program. Design, ornamentation and detailing are all for nothing if the structure will not last. So it is with fitness. Both require a sound foundation.

Floor work: The foundation

Many people are under the false impression that Pilates is a fitness program done on machines. However, the original Pilates Method, called *"Contrology,"* as presented in his book, **Return To Life**, is what is known today as the Pilates mat. In the *21st Century Fitness* formula, the number of exercises has been reduced from Pilates' original 34 to just 21 in order to save time. My students and I have demonstrated that this alteration to the Pilates method is effective.

The floor work is the foundation of the *21st Century Fitness* formula, and the missing link in most fitness programs. It exercises to full extension the majority of the muscles in the body, and it consists of precise and connected head-to-toe movements designed with economy of motion to stretch and strengthen muscle with resistance. This resistance is supplied by the body itself in the form of gravity. It is the stretch with resistance that gives alignment and builds the powerhouse muscles, which when stretched, stabilize the torso and strengthen the muscles so that they eventually hold their new, longer configuration.

Resistance is the difference between *21st Century Fitness* floor work and the traditional stretching methods taught in most exercise programs where the muscles return to their pre-stretched positions because they lack the resistance factor.

The floor work exercises create an awareness of the deep torso muscles. The exercises re-pattern muscular-skeletal imbalances and reintegrate the body. They are structured in such a way as to balance strength and flexibility, and to also increase the range of motion of the joints with greater strength and coordination. These exercises require concentration; they work the mind and body. They focus on "core" or "powerhouse" muscles: the abdomen, back and buttocks. Deep breathing is a very important component, and when done rhythmically, it is aerobic. As one becomes more proficient with the exercises and can perform the movements in flowing succession, there will be a noticeable increase in heart rate.

The first mark of identifying fitness is straightness. Stand tall! Posture is not an intellectual exercise, nor is it posing. Excellent posture comes from specific exercises and movements that align and position the body so that it stands tall naturally, not from thinking about standing tall. Very few people are given the gift of good posture; it must be developed. Floor work, in addition to the other elements in the *21st Century Fitness* formula, offers individuals the capability to stand tall naturally. These exercises do not put force on ligaments and joints, but only on the muscles that support them. Floor work can also be helpful during pregnancy and after childbirth to restore abdominal strength and realign posture.

Objectives of Floor Work: the foundation of
21st Century Fitness

1. Developing a straight spine and developing excellent posture
2. Developing flexibility and agility
3. Massaging the spine
4. Systematically massaging the various muscles of the body
5. Working the abdomen to develop the powerhouse
6. Stretching the hamstrings and legs
7. Strengthening the core body muscles
8. Opening the chest and enhancing breathing capabilities
9. Creating a leaner, taller body

ANTI - AGING AT ITS BEST

Fill-in Exercises

Fill-in exercises do just that: they "fill in" the gaps not covered by floor work, weight resistance and walking. There are only four fill-ins, and they can be done at almost any convenient time, whether at work, in school, or in some cases while talking on the phone. But the fill-ins are essential to the program and are not to be treated as after-thoughts.

Weight Resistance

My years of experience in weight training led me to conclude that this was an important component when done in combination with the floor work. Although weight resistance is isolated movement as opposed to connected movement, it magnifies and reinforces the benefits of floor work—-but only if done selectively! Too much weight training can erase the positive benefits of both. The **balance** is critical. Examples of the results we are trying to avoid are:

Back-neck presses, which overbuild and tighten the trapezoid muscles, causing the head to pitch forward and lock into place, compounding an inevitable aspect of aging.

Squats and lunges, which are hard on the joints and cause cumulative damage over the years, and also they can cause a curve to the lower back. With squats there is a tendency to over-build the muscles, creating a dispro-portion. Similar disproportions occur in other areas of the body when exercise movements are concentrated on single or small groups of muscles. By eliminating these and many other exercises associated with weight resist-ance, the critical balance is achieved and sleek (as opposed to bulky) muscles are developed.

With our weight resistance it is important to follow the recommendation as accurately as possible. You will not get the fast "pump up" that you get from conventional methods, adding more and more weights with fewer repe-titions. The *21st Century Fitness* formula takes longer, but it produces a more natural strength and a more natural appearance.

Walking

The importance of walking cannot be over-emphasized, from both the men-tal and the physical points of view. Walking is exhilarating. It clears the mind. It is excellent for your sense of mental well being, and it's excellent for the *metabolism*. It speeds up the chemical changes in living cells that pro-vide energy for vital processes like digestion. Walking uses the energy from food intake rather than storing that energy in the form of fat, and thus pro-vides the benefits of exercise in tandem with the benefits of good nutrition. Walking is also important for the shaping and strengthening of the hips and legs. It is the long aerobic complement to the short aerobics of floor work.

Nutrition

Nutrition and exercise go hand in hand: fuel in, energy out. Together they form the "engine" of the body and the basis for all other activities. We refer to the overall process as **metabolism**, and the speed at which the body performs such involuntary activities as breathing, heart rate, circulation, and digestion as the **metabolic rate**.

The Blueprint Completed

It is the combination of these building blocks of the **21st Century Fitness** formula — **floor work, weight resistance, walking, fill-ins and nutrition** — that provides you with the new dimension of fitness and will enable you at any age to retain or regain all *8 Essentials of Fitness*.

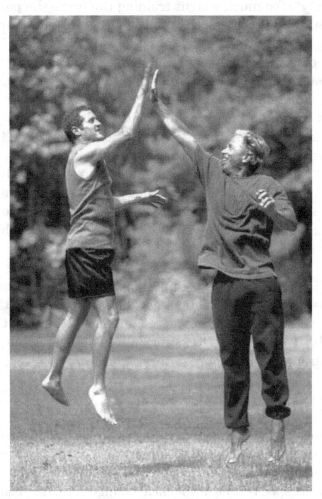

Chuck and Scott

Both Winners!

21st Century Fitness: Into Action

> **WHY SETTLE FOR LESS?**
> If you are going to spend the time and
> energy to exercise, you might as well
> obtain all *8 Essentials of Fitness.*

21st Century Fitness is a lifetime journey. There is no need to hurry. Be patient. Repetition is the key to success, and your goal is progress, not perfection. Perfection will come by carefully following the directions for each exercise and then repeating the exercises on a regular basis. You will meet success. To some it will come sooner, and to others it will come later, depending on your condition at the outset.

Before You Begin

Before starting any new exercise program it is wise to consult with your physician. If you are over 50, this consultation is strongly recommended. Pregnant women who have not done the Pilates mat or the *21st Century Fitness* floor work should not begin this program until after childbirth. However, the floor work can be helpful in maintaining fitness during pregnancy, and afterwards it helps to quickly restore abdominal strength and realign posture.

A note of caution: don't exercise immediately after eating; don't exercise when you're sick; don't exercise when you're overly tired.

Floor Work

Relax! Have fun! **Think of floor work as a sport**, and as with any sport, skill is achieved through practice and repetition. Do only the recommended number of exercises for each week of the program, and you will actually enjoy attaining *21st Century Fitness*. Don't worry if you're not moving along as fast as you think you should; I've never had a student who didn't "get it."

Each position of the body as shown in the diagrams—-the legs, the neck, the feet, etc.—-is very important. Please do not take shortcuts. There is a reason for every subtlety: each position, and each small movement in that position, is critical to the whole. If one or more of the details is overlooked or omitted, the usefulness of the exercise is compromised. The mastery of these subtleties is what allows for continuous improvement and growth. Remember: *21st Century Fitness* is not a "quick-fix". It is a program for life.

Getting Started

Rest only as necessary, as endurance becomes increasingly more important. Your goal for the end of week 25 is to do all the floor work without resting, thus achieving a highly aerobic workout. Breathe deeply and naturally. Where many regimens require specific methods of breathing, the *21st Century Fitness* formula does not. Move smoothly and gracefully. Movements that are sped up or jerky should be avoided, but this does not mean slow motion!

If you are not strong enough in the beginning to do any of the following exercises shown (long roll up, stretch forward, criss cross stretch, etc.), tuck your feet under a chair or sofa for added support. Or, you can purchase 5-lb. ankle weights and lay them flat over your ankles. Many conventional fitness programs advise against doing sit-up type exercises with legs straight. The *21st Century Fitness* formula sit-up exercises, because of their subtleties — leading with the head, curving the spine going both backward and forward — do allow for straight legs.

Start slowly. Use a rug or mat. As you progress you will learn the exercises. We deliberately begin with only five exercises and add new ones at a slow pace for these reasons: (1) to avoid strain (2) to accustom the muscles and bone structure to new positions (3) so that you will memorize the exercises as you move ahead. No matter what your age or physical condition, you are cautioned to perform these exercises at the rates and schedules indicated. Please do not speed up!

When you are experienced at the floor work, you will do the entire routine in 20-25 minutes. Until you have gained experience, and even though you will begin with far fewer exercises (as the floor work table indicates), you will need the full 20-25 minutes to memorize and learn the techniques. After week 25 you are on your own to continue ahead at your own pace.

> **Look for miracles! The *21st Century Fitness* formula floor work, the foundation of the program, will enable your body to do things you never dreamed possible.**

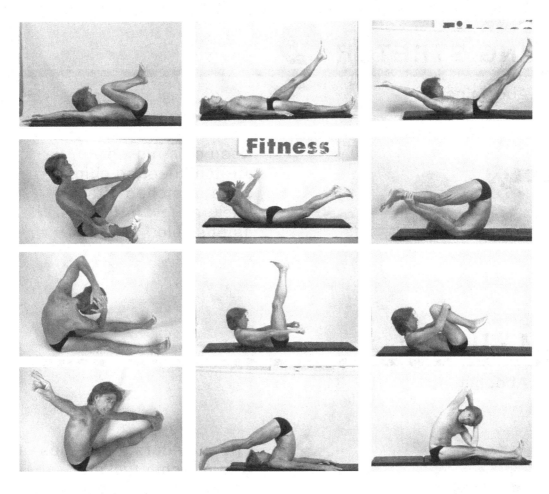

Larry pictured doing Floor Work at age 75
The test of Agility, Flexibility, and Strength.

FLOOR WORK (1 THROUGH 21)

1. Opening Stretch
2. Warm Up
3. Legs Up
4. Long Roll Up
5. Leg Shaper
6. The Roll
7. Single-Leg Slide
8. Double-Leg Slide
9. Spine Stretch
10. V-Roll

11. The Tower
12. Leg Circles
13. Windmill
14. Reverse Kick
15. Body Surfer
16. Stretch Forward
17. Criss-cross Stretch
18. Ballet
19. Swim
20. B-29
21. Release

ANTI - AGING AT ITS BEST

OPENING STRETCH ❶

Focus: Abdominals

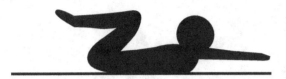

❶ Keep chin tucked,
stretch knees to chin,
arms stretched straight
back, as low to floor
as possible.

WARM - UP ❷

Focus: Abdominals

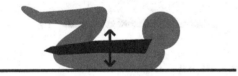

❶ Lift shoulders 3-4 inches off
ground, chin tucked.
Stretch knees towards chin,
arms extended 2 inches
from floor, pump arms
up and down briskly. Hands
to stop 2 inches off floor.
Feet relaxed.

LEG - UP ❸

Focus: Abdominals, Hamstring stretch

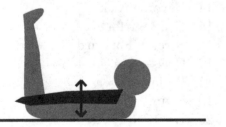

❶ Continue as in #2 (warm-up).
Keep chin tucked, extend
legs at right angle, feet relaxed.

ROLL - UP 4 Use ankle weights across feet if needed.

Focus: Shin muscles, Upper back muscles, Stretch to Latisimus

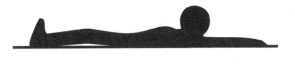

1 Lying on your back, flex your feet, arms stretched behind head and flat on floor.

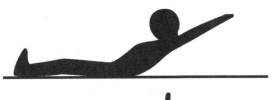

2 Roll up and stretch for toes, Lead with head, arms travel with head.

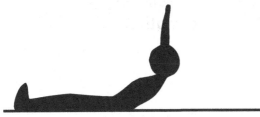

3

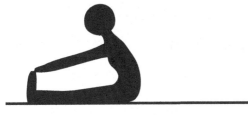

4

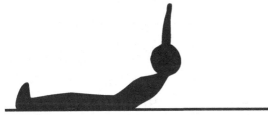

5 Slowly roll back into starting position. Curve spine, lower vertebrae by vertebrae.

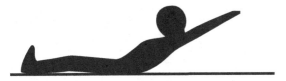

6

7 Return to flat position.

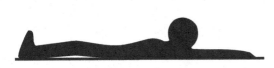

27

LEG SHAPER ⑤

Focus: Hip flexors, knee extensors

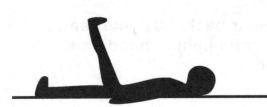

1 Lying on your back, arms at sides, head and neck flat, with feet relaxed.

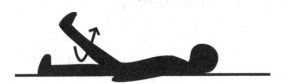

2 Bring leg straight down into a counter clockwise motion.

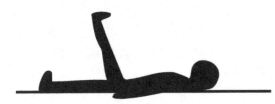

3 Pause at top, repeat 8x.

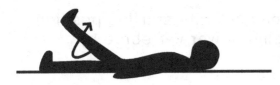

4 Reverse motion and repeat 8x.

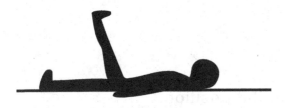

5 Repeat other leg.

THE ROLL **6**

Focus: Abdominals, dynamic postural control, balance

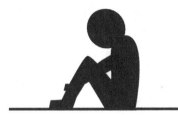

1 Keep chin and body tucked, feet relaxed.

2 Roll body backward to floor.

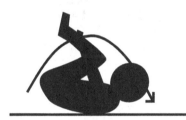

3

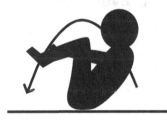

4 Roll forward.

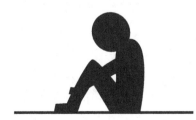

5 Return to starting position, without touching feet to the floor.

ANTI - AGING AT ITS BEST

SINGLE-LEG SLIDE

Focus: Stretch to hip extensors with knee to chest, work to abdominals hip flexors with leg extended.

2 Keep chin tucked, feet relaxed. Roll shoulders off mat, pull knee to chin with outside hand holding knee, inside hand holding ankle. Extended leg remains off floor at approximately 50°.

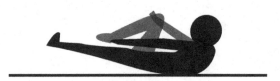

3 Alternate knee to chest while keeping extended leg at 50° to prevent back strain.

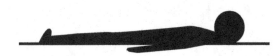

4

DOUBLE-LEG SLIDE 8

Focus: Abdominals, hip flexors

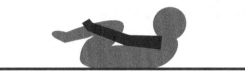

1 Keep chin tucked, feet relaxed.

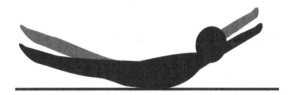

2 While extending arms and legs, raise shoulders off mat, keep legs approximately 50° from floor. Simultaneously stretch arms and legs.
Do not lower head or shoulders.
Do not extend arms lower than head.

3

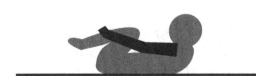

ANTI - AGING AT ITS BEST

SPINE STRETCH ⑨

Focus: Stretch to hamstrings and trunk and neck extensors

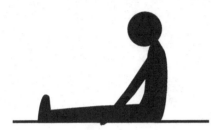

❶ Feet shoulder width and flexed.

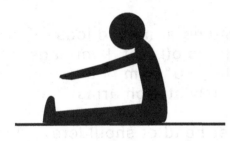

❷ Leading with head, reach for toes.

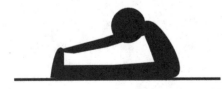

❸ Bring head as close to knees as possible, touch toes and hold for 10 counts. Relax. Return to sitting position and start #10 V-ROLL.

V-ROLL Advanced (Do not execute until after week 11)

Focus: Abdominals and dynamic postural control

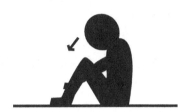

1 Eyes down, feet relaxed, legs separated. Hold calves under knees. Legs create a "V" as you roll back

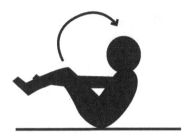

2 Start roll.

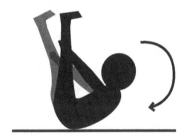

3 Roll back to floor exending legs into a " V ".

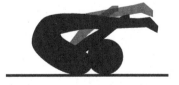

4 Keep eyes down.

Anti - Aging at its best

V-ROLL - (continued)

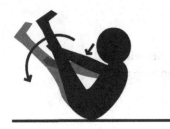

5 Roll legs forward and look at crotch.

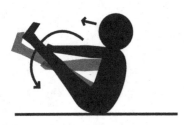

6 When bottom hits floor look straight ahead and anchor eyes. Hold for 5 counts. Stretch legs and open chest. Feet do not touch floor.

7 Roll back.

8 Repeat.

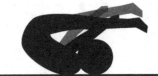

TOWER ⓫ Advanced (Do not execute until after week 25)

Focus: Abdominals, posterior deltoids, rhomboids, trapezoids

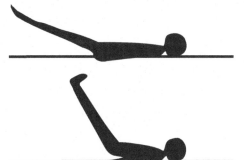

❶

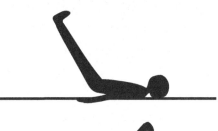

❷ Keep legs together, bring over head.

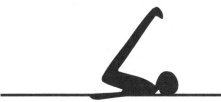

❸ Raise hips and lower trunk off mat.

❹ Roll backward, touch toes to floor.

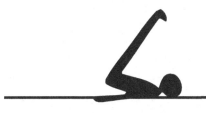

❺ Come forward.
Keep head flat on floor.
Hands on floor for balance.
Do not arch neck.

❻ Anchor lower back to floor.

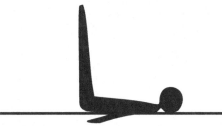

❼ Lower legs to a few inches
off the floor.

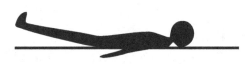

❽ Make a counter clockwise half circle,
do not touch legs to floor.

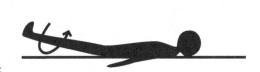

TOWER - (continued)

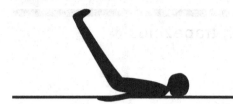

9 Come back up and repeat.

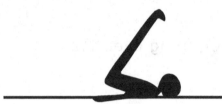

10

11

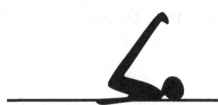

12

13

14

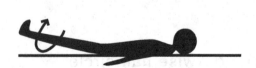

15 Make a clockwise circle, do not touch legs to floor.

LEG CIRCLES Advanced (Do not execute until after week 25)

Focus: Abdominals, hip flexors

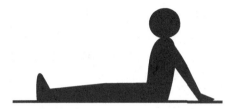

1 Feet together and relaxed. Arms as straight as possible anchored on floor.

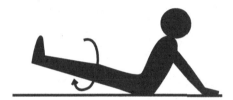

2 Lift legs straight up and and over in a clockwise motion, in a " D " formation.

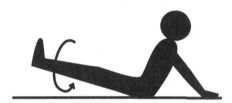

3 Pause at top of each cicle, do not touch legs to floor. Repeat in a counter clockwise rotation.

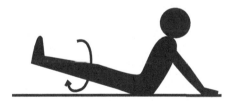

4

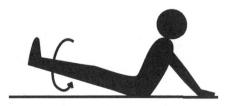

5

WINDMILL 13

Focus: Stretch to hamstrings and trunk

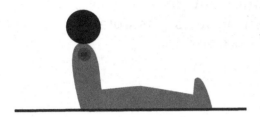

1 Arms straight out to side, keep palms up. Sit up as straight as possible, feet flexed.

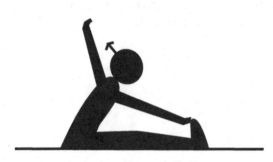

2 Touch pinky finger to little toe of opposite foot, eyes look to raised palm.

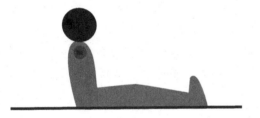

3 Return to center, pause, sit up straight, and look straight ahead.

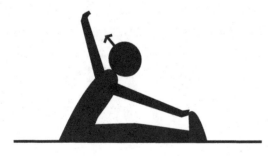

4 Repeat to opposite side.

REVERSE KICK

Focus: Hamstrings with trunk and neck extensors

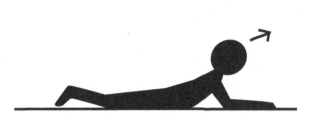

1 Lying on stomach, keep fists pressed against floor, shoulder width apart and straight up. Feet relaxed slightly off floor. Keep eyes to ceiling.

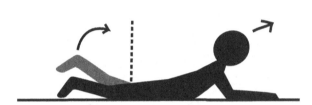

2 Bend leg at knee into a right angle, kick twice.

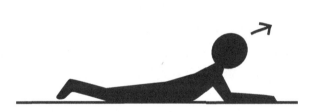

3 Return. Do not touch foot to floor (keep about 2 inches off floor).

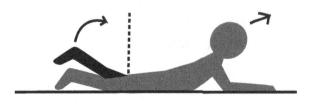

4 Repeat with opposite leg. Remember: do not touch feet to floor.

ANTI - AGING AT ITS BEST

BODY SURFER Advanced (Do not execute until after week 16)

Focus: Trunk, leg, and arm extensors; stretch to abdominals

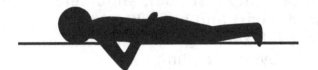

1 Clasp hands behind lower back, head faces left. Feet relaxed.

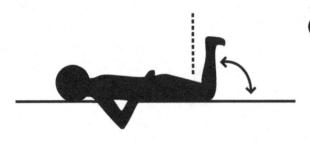

2 Keep hands clasped behind back. Bend knees into a right angle and kick 3 x.

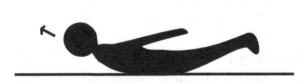

3 Raise head, upper torso and legs, and straighten arms. Eyes stretched to ceiling. Return to first position with head facing right. Repeat reversing head position.

STRETCH FORWARD ⓰ Use ankle weights if needed.

Focus: Abdominal with stretch to back muscles; trunk extensors with stretch to abdominals.

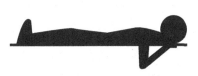
1 Feet flexed and shoulder width apart. Hands clasped under head.

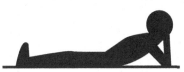
2 Leading with head roll up off floor

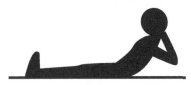
3

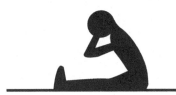
4

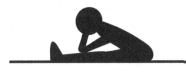
5 Stretch elbows to knees.

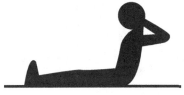
6 Stretch straight up and out of hips and sit up.

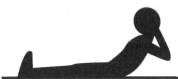
7 Roll back vertebrae by vertebrae.

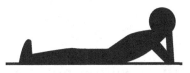
8

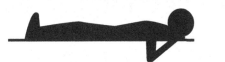
9

CRISS - CROSS KNEE STRETCH

Focus: Abdominal and hip flexors, stretch to hamstrings and trunk

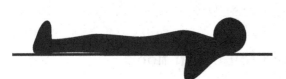

1 Feet flexed, shoulder width apart.

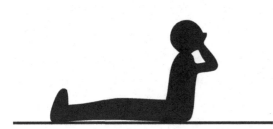

2 Stretch straight up and out of hips. Sit up.

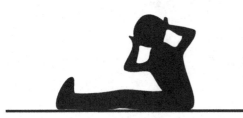

3 Rotate opposite elbow to opposite knee.

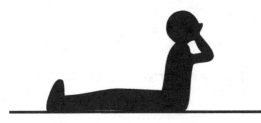

4 Stretch straight up and out of hips and sit up.

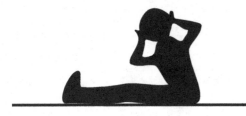

5 Repeat positions 3 and 4 with other side. Then roll back to position 1 vertebrae by vertebrae.

42

BALLET 18 Advanced (Do not execute until after week 25)

Focus: Abdominals, stretch to back, dynamic balance, upper trunk and shoulder extensors, anterior tibialis, hamstring and calf stretch

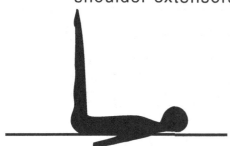

1 Arms to sides, legs extended feet relaxed.

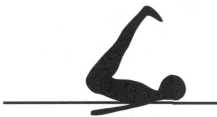

2 Roll back and stretch legs to ceiling.

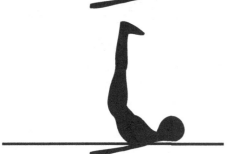

3 Flex feet and stretch heels to ceiling.

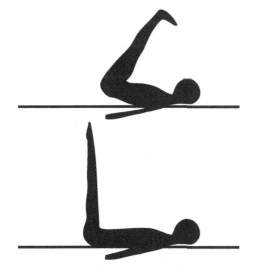

4 Roll down vertebrae by vertebrae. Continue stretching heels until lower back reaches floor. Keep neck flat to floor.

5 Legs should form right angle, relax feet and repeat.

SWIM **19**

Focus: Arm, trunk, and leg extensors

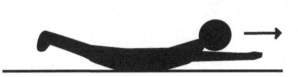

1 Lying on stomach, extend arms and legs. Eyes raised to ceiling. Feet relaxed.

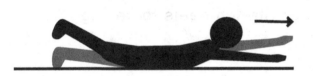

2 Proceed with a swimming motion opposite leg with opposite arm.

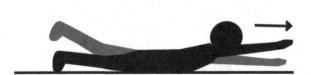

3

B-29 **20**

Focus: Middle shoulder muscles, arm extensors, trunk and leg extensors, stretch to chest.

1 Lying on stomach, head faces left, arms extended to sides, toes pointed.

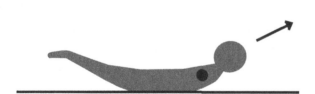

2 Lift arms, legs and head into air arching back. Eyes raised to ceiling.

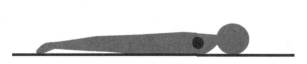

3 Reverse head and repeat.

RELEASE ㉑

Focus: Abdominals, dynamic balance

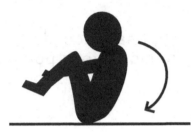

1 Keep chin and body tucked, feet apart. Arms inside thighs grasping ankles.

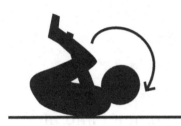

2 Roll back until shoulders touch floor. Tap feet twice.

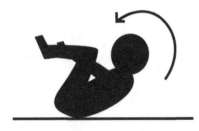

3 Roll forward.

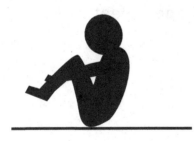

4 When feet are approximately 3 inches off the ground, tap twice.

Table of Floor Work Exercises

Maximum Repetitions	Exercise	Weeks 1-4	Weeks 5-10	Weeks 11-15	Weeks 16-24	Weeks 25 & Beyond
	Opening Stretch	X	X	X	X	X
25	Warm-Up	X	X	X	X	X
75	Legs-Up		X	X	X	X
15	Long Roll-Up			X	X	X
8	Leg Shaper (ea. leg)		X	X	X	X
6	The Roll	X	X	X	X	X
30	Single Leg Slide	X	X	X	X	X
30	Double Leg Slide		X	X	X	X
1	Spine Stretch	X	X	X	X	X
8	V-Roll			X	X	X
6	The Tower					X
8	Leg Circles					X
10	Windmill			X	X	X
50	Reverse Kick			X	X	X
5	Body Surfer				X	X
8	Stretch Forward			X	X	X
12	Criss-cross Stretch				X	X
5	Ballet					X
75	Swim			X	X	X
6	B-29			X	X	X
6	Release		X	X	X	X

Caution: Do only as many repetitions of an exercise that is comfortable. The amount of repetitions noted are the maximum to be accomplished over time, so its okay to start with 1 or 2. Do not strain! No rush!

Fill-in Exercises

Fill-in exercises do just that—-they "fill in" the gaps not covered by the floor work, weight resistance and walking. They are designed to give extra attention to specific areas of the body that resist change. Examples of these areas are "love handles," the "belly" and "saddlebags". There are only four fill-ins and they can be done at any convenient time: at work, in school, and. in some cases, while talking on the phone. There is no particular order in which they should be performed, but they are essential to the program and not to be treated as afterthoughts.

Getting Started

Breathe naturally. With the abdominal exercises, start at 5 repetitions and progress to 100. With the Butt Pinches, start at 20 repetitions and progress to 150. Toe Raises: females start at 10 repetitions and progress to 50 (to provide shape rather than muscularity). Males start at 10 and progress to 100. Arm Circles: start at 10 and 10 (forward and backward) and progress to 50 and 50. If initially you don't feel your muscles connecting, just continue. It might take a month or two, so don't be discouraged.

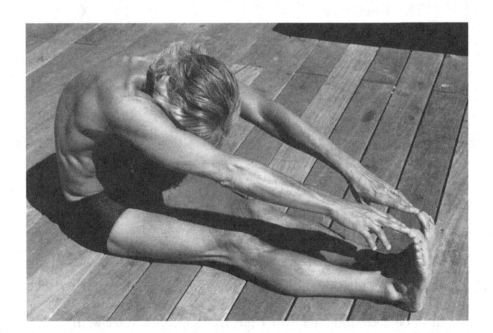

BUTT PINCH

Focus: Upper shoulder muscles, stretch to latisimus, buttocks

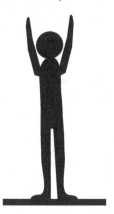

1 Stretch arms above head.
Rapidly clench and release
buttocks muscle.
Feet shoulder width and
look straight ahead.

TOE RAISE

Focus: Calf muscles

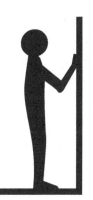

1 Stand with hands
against wall.

2 Press up lifting
heels and return
to floor.
Use arms for
balance only.

ARM CIRCLE

Focus: Shoulder muscles, strengten latisimus

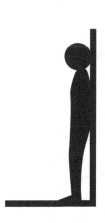

1 Stand with back
against wall, arms
extended, feet
shoulder width.

Feet 10-12 inches
from wall.

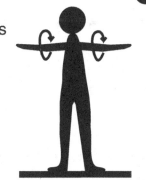

2 Rotate arms in a
clockwise motion.
Repeat with a
counterclockwise
motion.

RAINBOW

Focus: Shoulder muscles, upper shoulder muscles, stretch to latisimus.

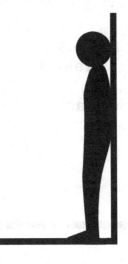

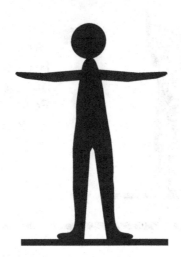

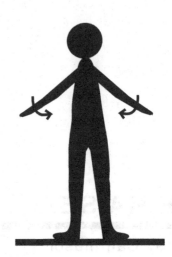

1 Stand with small of back against wall. Press head to wall. Feet 10-12" from wall. Knees slightly bent.

2 Extend arms to sides at a right angle.

3 Swing arms downward with palms down.

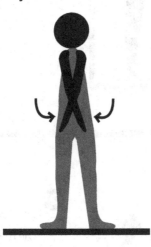

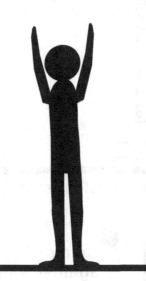

4 Extend arms fully downward.

5 Move both arms straight forward in upward direction until fully stretched toward ceiling through fingertips. Do not release back or head from wall, eyes straight forward. Repeat 2x.

RAINBOW- (continued)

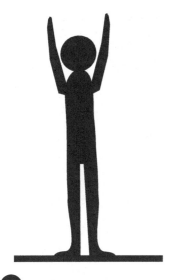

6 Move arms forward and straight down.

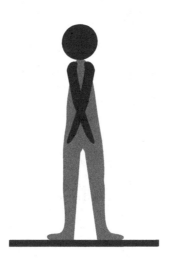

7 Extend arms fully downward.

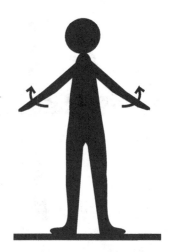

8 Swing arms sideward and upward.

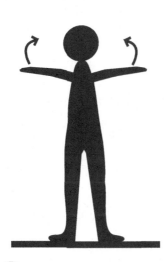

9 Swing both arms out and up over head, palms up.

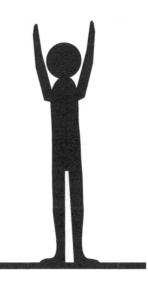

10 Fully straighten both arms to ceiling through fingertips. Do not release back or head from wall, eyes straight forward. Repeat 2x.

ABDOMINALS

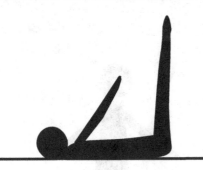

1 Position legs at a right angle. Reach up toward toes as high as possible.

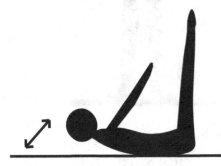

2 Return to floor and repeat.

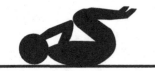

1 Feet together, knees slightly apart.

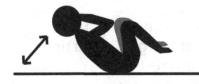

2 Stretch forward with both elbows and reach over both knees. Pull back and repeat.

Anti - Aging at its best

ABDOMINALS

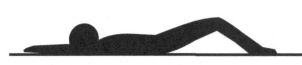

1 Knees shoulder width apart and bent.

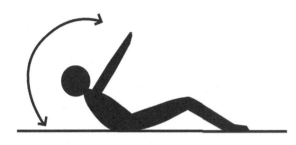

2 Stretch forward, roll back, repeat.

ADVANCED (Do not execute until after week 20)

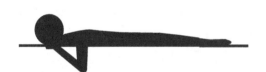

1

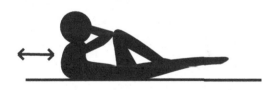

2 Stretch forward and touch right knee to right elbow, stretch back (as arrow indicates). Keep extended leg slightly off floor.

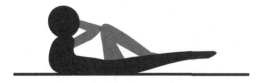

3 Come forward.
Repeat with left side.

ANTI - AGING AT ITS BEST

Weight Resistance

Weight resistance is very critical to the **21st Century Fitness** formula. It is the fine-tuning. You will note that these five simple exercises are only for the upper body. The floor work, toe raises and walking provide all most people need for the legs. Beyond this fine-tuning, weight resistance exercises are to be avoided because many are detrimental to the goals of the **21st Century Fitness** formula. For instance, squats and lunges work against the straightness of the spine, build muscle bulk, tighten muscles, and are hard on the joints. All of these work against the objective of achieving the essentials of youth in our later years.

Getting Started

Breathe deeply and naturally. Always stretch arms out fully; partial extension creates short, bulky muscles. Remember, long and lean is the goal.

Keep weights light and aim for more repetitions. Heavier weights result in bulk. Dumbbells for men should be between 10 and 20 lbs. each; never go beyond 20. For women they should be between 3 and 10 lbs. each, and never go beyond 10. Start at a comfortable weight and go the maximum indicated.

Feet should be placed shoulder width apart and facing a wall straight on. Look into a mirror if available. For balance and optimum body position, keep eyes focused straight ahead, never up and down.

Never hyper-extend knees; they should always be slightly bent. Continue to add weight until maximum weight and repetition are achieved. Remember: no rush. Relax.

Repetitions

	MEN	WOMEN
Press	15 - 20	10 - 12
Curl *	15 - 20	10 - 12
Chin Press	15 - 20	10 - 12
Shrug	40 - 50	20 - 30
Back/Neck	30 - 50	10 - 20

*Each Arm

PRESS

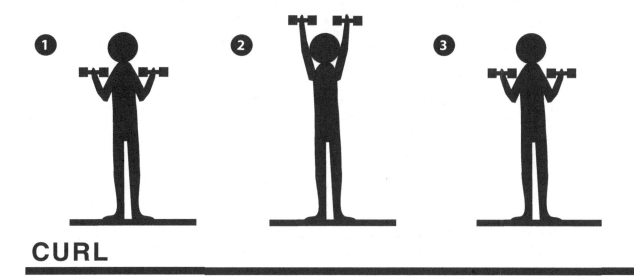

CURL

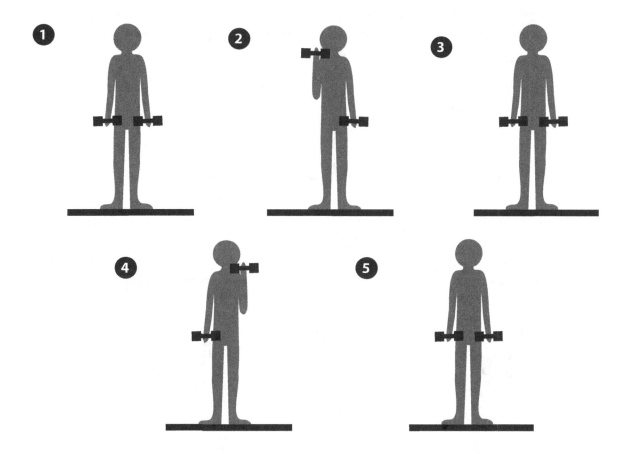

CHIN PRESS

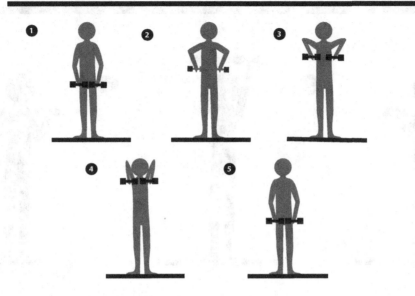

SHOULDER SHRUG

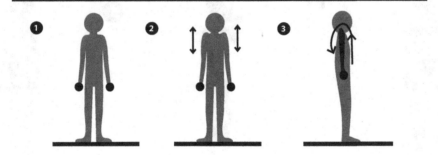

BACK NECK PRESS

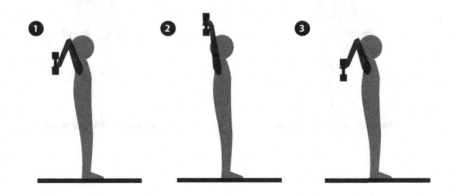

Walking

While 20 minutes of floor work is an aerobic workout, you will rely on walking as your main aerobic exercise. It is also the key to your leg and hip work and should be done without stopping. According to Joseph Pilates, "The art of correct walking consists primarily and simply in a slight tilting forward of the proper standing posture."

Walk straight, head high, eyes forward. The object is to feel the back of the upper leg and the butt stretching. Do not lean forward. Walking reinforces stomach strength and **Standing Tall**.

Starting at a comfortable pace, build up to a maximum walking speed of 3.5 to 4.5 miles per hour. Arms should swing forward and backward comfortably. There are those who suggest various arm positions, but as with natural breathing in all exercises, I suggest a natural position for your arms when walking.

WALKING

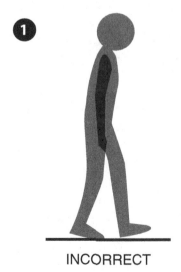

INCORRECT

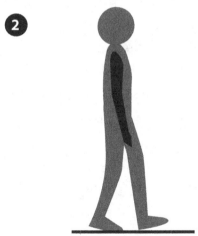

CORRECT

Nutrition

Exercise alone will not get you fit. You also need proper nutrition. It is an essential aspect of the *21st Century Fitness* formula to become *8 Essential Fit*. (See Nutrition Supplement, pg. 108)

Sleep

While not an element of the *21st Century Fitness* formula, I include sufficient sleep as another important, but frequently overlooked, necessity for fitness. Sleep rejuvenates the body. All available research indicates that your sleep requirements do not diminish as you grow older, especially if you are getting proper exercise. It is recommended that you complete your exercise routines at least two hours before you go to bed. Exercise raises the body's core temperature, which doesn't begin to drop off significantly until about two hours later. When timed properly, exercise will prolong a deeper sleep (called "slow wave" sleep) during the first hour of nighttime rest. It is also recommended that you not go to bed hungry. (See suggestions in Nutrition Chapter)

Objectives of the *21st Century Fitness* Formula

- Massage, align and stretch the spine
- Improve posture
- Systematically stretch and exercise the "whole" body
- Improve muscle tone
- Develop the powerhouse muscles
- Strengthen the legs
- Stretch the hamstrings
- Work the biceps and triceps
- Stretch the inner and outer thighs
- Strengthen the neck
- Elongate the calf muscles
- Strengthen the heart and lungs
- Improve breathing
- Improve flexibility and agility
- Increase energy
- Build definition and proportion
- Release tension

Scheduling

Scheduling is imperative. Like most rules, schedules will be broken, but setting a schedule will serve to remind you to make up lost sessions by creating a gap (on paper or in your mind) when your schedule is disrupted. You should schedule each of your *21st Century Fitness* formula components, but the formula offers generous make-goods on schedule disruptions.

If You Miss It, Make It Up

You can do your workouts in broken sessions. For example, fill-ins can be done separately on the same day, one full-hour session can make up for a lost day, or you can separate your daily workout with part in the morning and the rest done during your lunch or in the evening. There is an endless variety of "chip away" combinations; that is one of the great advantages of always having your program with you. (One useful tip: keep your dumbbells near your TV.) Flexibility is the key, and while you can break up the resistance and fill-ins, floor work and walking should be completed without interruption.

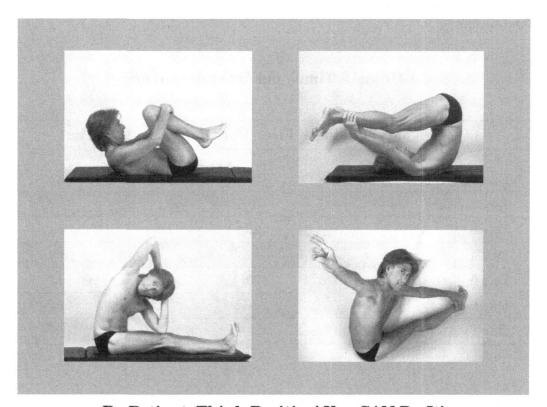

Be Patient. Think Positive! You CAN Do It!

ANTI - AGING AT ITS BEST

30-Minute Per Day Regimen (average)

	Weight	Walking	Floor Work	Fill-ins	Time
Day 1	(20)				20 min.
Day 2			(20)	(10)	30 min.
Day 3	(20)	(20)			40 min.
Day 4			(20)	(10)	30 min.
Day 5	(20)	(20)			40 min.
Day 6			(20)	(10)	30 min.
Day 7		(20)			20 min.

Note: Weight resistance must be done with one day of rest between sessions. Walking can be done at any time of day, three times per week. Alternate days are OK, but not necessary. The same applies for floor work and fill-ins.

1 Hour: 3 Times per Week Regimen

	Weight	Walking	Floor Work	Fill-ins	Time
Day 1	(20)	(20)	(20)	(10)	70 min
Day 2					
Day 3	(20)	(20)	(20)	(10)	70 min.
Day 4					
Day 5	(20)	(20)	(20)	(10)	70 min.
Day 6					
Day 7					

Anti - Aging at its best

Mental Preparation

Intent and action are often confused. Action, not intent, achieves results. The key to success is taking the first step, adhering to your schedule and following the instructions. It's that simple. Once you get the rhythm it will be as comfortable as an old shoe. See yourself there. Focus on becoming *8 Essential Fit. Believe it to be attainable.* My students and I are living proof. Do not let yourself become distracted by the myriad of exercise programs and diets. Be patient. Allow the ***21st Century Fitness*** formula the time to work for you.

NO JOGGING!!!

No Jogging is the No Smoking of the 21st Century.

**Jogging after 35 speeds up the effect of gravity.
As we age, the goal is to defy gravity.**

Jogging is also hard on the joints; and the goal is to protect our joints so they will last and not require replacement. The solution is walking. You will get the same benefits without the wear and tear.

And to always remember —

**THE PURPOSE OF MODERN FITNESS
IS TO STAY YOUNG!**

The Steps to *21st Century Fitness*

1. Surrender - be willing to change.

2. Take responsibility for your own physical well being. Fitness is more than just another choice. Give *21st Century Fitness* a priority value in your life.

3. Realize you have to do something. Premature aging comes to everyone who fails to take action.

4. Accept the fact that quick-fix methods do not work.

5. Take Action. Follow the formula. Don't waver. Live with *21st Century Fitness*. Don't be "creative."

6. Provide yourself with continuous re-enforcement by re-reading this book.

7. See yourself there: *8 Essential Fit*.

8. Relax. Think of it as a sport.

9. Expect a perpetual state of well-being.

10. Be patient. Give the miracle time to happen.

21st Century Fitness Prevention

In our society there tends to be a prevailing attitude that if you show a serious interest in your physical condition, especially in regard to exercise and nutrition, you are a "health nut." However, in other cultures the health conscious are viewed as enlightened people with strength of character, strong convictions and wisdom.

Furthermore, in America we generally don't worry about our health until we get sick. Then we go to our doctors and expect them to cure us; we are not prevention-minded. In our passive concern for preserving our health and preventing disease we have become medically-dependent.

Now at the dawn of the 21st Century, despite all of our medical advances, more Americans than ever are dying of cancer, heart disease and stroke. According to the latest figures, 33% of us will develop some form of cancer, and 50% of us will develop some form of cardiovascular disease. In many cases these diseases can be prevented.

In addition to the preventable killers, we Americans are also suffering from degenerative diseases and conditions such as osteoporosis, arthritis, malaise, and lack of mobility. While not necessarily fatal, they do cause widespread misery, yet most people consider them normal aspects of the aging process because they most often occur in those over 50. More and more doctors, however, believe these diseases and conditions can be prevented by changes in lifestyle, and especially through intelligent nutrition.

Oxidation

The process by which the body converts food to energy is called oxidation. This conversion produces by-products, much the way a fire causes ashes, and these are called free radicals. Your body produces them not only from the metabolism of food and exercise, but also from the inhalation of smoke and polluted air, and from sun-exposure. Oxidation and the production of free radicals occurs throughout your life, and over time these by-products cause parts of your body to degenerate. Free radicals in your joints, for example, are a cause of arthritis. In your skin free radicals cause wrinkles as well as various forms of skin cancer. In your blood vessels they cause strokes. Since oxidation is a natural process, and the free radicals it produces are unavoidable, there is a way to combat their degenerative effects: fruits and vegetables.

An ounce of prevention is worth a pound of cure

ANTI - AGING AT ITS BEST

The Old Folks Were Right

Fruits and vegetables help to fight the effects of free radicals because, in addition to providing an array of nutrients, these foods contain anti-oxidants such as Vitamin C, beta carotene and others which have specific affects on certain organs. Lycopene in tomatoes, for example, according to the American Cancer Society, is helpful in reducing the risk of prostate cancer.

But this isn't news at all! Your parents and grandparents might be remembered for such seemingly inane comments as, "Rabbits never wear glasses," when they directed you to eat your vegetables. Now, the discovery of oxidation and its resulting free radicals becomes a sudden wake-up call to the truth of those directives: those older people knew what they were talking about!

Dr. Alan Cott of New York City was one of America's earliest physicians to devote his entire practice to nutrition and food supplements. He stressed the importance of fruits, vegetables and anti-oxidants in the treatment of people of all ages for a variety of conditions and diseases. I had the good fortune to be a longtime patient of Dr. Cott, and I realized, while formulating *21st Century Fitness*, that the nutrition portion of the program needed the same intense scrutiny I was giving to the exercise regimen. I have integrated the teachings of Dr. Cott with my own studies and experience to formulate a dietary plan designed to fulfill all objectives of nutrition. The goals of this plan go far beyond cosmetics. The focus of *21st Century Fitness* nutrition is prevention and good health. My students and I are living testaments to the validity of combining the exercises and nutrition of the formula, and the importance of incorporating both to become *8 Essential Fit*.

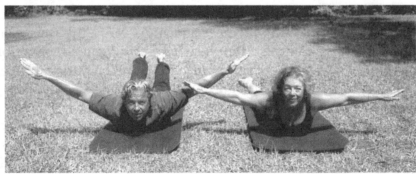

Scott Settle   *Carole Settle*

Most "diets" fail because they don't build a high level of antioxidents. There is no doubt the pounds will come off but will the level of antioxidents go up? We can't stay young without a high level of antioxidents.

ANTI - AGING AT ITS BEST

21st Century Fitness Nutrition

Americans are confused about nutrition. A well known magazine's survey reports that 55% are fed up with nutritionists' advice because they are getting conflicting information. 46% said they were confused by competitive product claims on food packages, leaving them unsure about what foods to eat. The greatest number - 77% - said they believe that in a short time the "experts" will have a completely different idea about which foods are healthful and which are not.

The confusion about nutrition is equaled by the confusion about exercise. Many people have some interest in nutrition and maintaining a fit body, but conflicting "research" has us reeling. We don't know what to do. And when we don't know what to do, generally we do nothing.

One thing the "experts" do agree on is that exercise and nutrition are mutually co-dependent in building fitness. Even the popular belief that exercise will offset or correct poor eating habits is quickly dispelled by simply pointing out that it takes an hour or more on a treadmill to burn just 300 calories.

If we begin with the basics, nutrition is de-mystified. The following are the objectives of nutrition that provide the guideposts to an understanding of our bodies needs.

Objectives of Nutrition

Build a Strong Metabolism

Provide Nourishment

Maximize Digestion

Maximize Energy

Balance the System

Minimize Mood Swings

Rebuild Tissue and Cells

Maximize Vitamin and Mineral Intake

Burn Fat Cells and Be Lean

Feel Good and Enjoy Long-Lasting Youth

Metabolism: The Foundation

The goal of **21st Century Fitness** nutrition is to permanently improve your metabolism with a balanced combination of exercise and nutrition so that you can eat normally without dieting. A healthy metabolism acts as an equalizer, and you will discover that it will allow you to lose or even gain weight naturally. Over time your body will discover its own optimum weight.

Finding Your Optimum Weight

The goal of nutrition is not to be thin, nor is it cosmetic. The goal is to accomplish the objectives of nutrition (covered on the previous page), and in doing so, to find your optimum weight. Optimum weight results from a healthy metabolism, and that results from effective nutrition and exercise: the right formula and the balance. **21st Century Fitness** "core" foods, when eaten at the right times, will result in your attaining and maintaining your optimum weight.

It is reasonably easy to get thin through diets, but in most cases the thinness is accomplished at the expense of the objectives of nutrition. The significant difference between the **21st Century Fitness** nutritional plan and typical fad diets is that with my plan you "eat yourself lean" with this balanced formula. Those who adopt an "of the moment" fad diet (the high protein diet is a good example) and make it to their weight loss goal have only gone part of the way. The trick is maintaining their new, lower weight.

There is no question that people who use a high-protein diet for weight loss can shed pounds, but the body does not store appreciable amounts of proteins. It uses what is needed, and the rest is then used for energy or stored in the form of fat. The problem is that animal proteins cause the buildup of certain toxins, causing self-poisoning, or autointoxication. To add to the problem, meat, with the exception of some organ meats, is a one-sided protein food, practically devoid of most vitamins and low in mineral content. And it is common knowledge that meat, no matter how lean, is loaded with saturated fats and cholesterol, which may cause heart disease.

A diet high in protein causes biochemical imbalances in the system, especially with respect to vitamins. Because in most cases carbohydrates from grains and fruit are minimal, or not included at all in these diets, the dieter is again missing the vitamins, minerals, enzymes and other vital substances essential to the body. Sooner or later we must regain the balance in our bodies and return to healthy ways of eating. It is the change in eating habits, combined with the metabolism being significantly out of balance that usually triggers relapse, and causes us to gain weight again.

It should now be clear that most fad diets, including the popular high protein diet, fail to take into consideration all 10 objectives of nutrition identified at the beginning of the chapter.

Key Principles of Nutrition

In the preceding chapter I discussed prevention. It is the combination of prevention and the right nutrition that enables us to reach our goal of long-lasting youth. The key principles in *21st Century Fitness* nutrition are:

Anti-oxidants

Natural Sugars

Low-fat

High Fiber

Minimal Salt

No Processed Flour

Eating the right foods at the right time

The combination of these principles provides you with the basis for a sound nutritional formula, and they will be your points of reference throughout the *21st Century Fitness* nutritional plan.

The Pleasure Principle

There is no question that eating affords one of life's great pleasures, and any fitness method that fails to acknowledge this basic fact of human nature is unrealistic. We all love to eat, and throughout history the richer civilizations and countries have fallen prey to over-indulgence in physical pleasure. None of those civilizations, however, have matched America's imbalance between over-eating and good nutrition. The *21st Century Fitness* nutritional plan is balanced. And it is forgiving, in the sense that it allows for the occasional over-indulgence through the pleasure principle without sacrificing any of the **Objectives of Nutrition.** If you are habitually eating the right foods, an occasional slab of red meat and calorie laden birthday cake is not going to throw your fitness into a tailspin.

Experience Is Our Guide

It is important to state that this nutritional plan is derived from experience: mine, my students and from what I have culled from widely acknowledged leaders in the field of nutrition, especially the late Dr. Alan Cott of New York City. I am not a nutritionist myself, nor am I a scientist, but I have experimented with a wide variety of nutritional plans over the years, and today my fitness reflects the best of those plans. While reasons for recommendations are frequently provided, I have taken the liberty of not attempting to scientifically explain every single one. The focus here is on the broad subject of nutrition, and the goal is simplicity.

Into Action

Anyone familiar with dietary trends will quickly recognize this nutrition plan as essentially Mediterranean in origin. The mainstays of diet in Mediterranean countries are generous servings of whole grain foods - bread, pasta, rice, polenta and couscous. Lots of fresh fruits and vegetables. Dairy products and meat play a secondary role as protein sources. Dried beans, nuts, lentils, chickpeas or pignoli combined with whole grain protein provides a complete protein diet, without much of the fat found in animal products.

Where the traditional American nutritional pyramid puts legumes, poultry, fish and red meat in the same category, the Mediterranean pyramid does not. Legumes are recommended for daily eating, chicken and fish for a few times a week, and lean red meat only a few times a month - if at all. (Please note that these recommendations are for healthy adults. Children require greater amounts of protein and fat.)

Nutritional Elements

In an architect's plan for a building there are certain elements of engineering that must be followed in order to assure integrity of construction. This is also true in regard to a plan for nutrition. The following are the elements of the *21st Century Fitness* nutritional formula:

• Upon rising, drink one cup of hot water with juice of a whole lemon. This cleanses the system, is a good source of Vitamin C and provides a burst of energy.

• Drink eight 8-ounce glasses of water daily. This also cleanses the system and provides the fluid required for cells and tissues.

• Eat slowly; talk a lot. Eating should be an enjoyable time of socializing, a tradition in every culture. Doing so aids digestion and controls appetite.

• Control fat intake to a maximum of 50 grams a day. The success of this regimen is based on fat intake. It requires an awareness of calories, but not fanatic counting. The base of your fat intake should be olive oil, flax seed oil, soy, almonds, fish and fowl.

• Eat three meals a day and two fruit snacks (one of them an apple) between meals. Apples are a good source of dietary fiber, including pectin, which helps lower cholesterol levels. One-half or a whole grapefruit an hour before retiring is optional. It, too, cleanses the body with soluble fiber, which again helps lower cholesterol, and it is also a good source of potassium.

• Do not mix fruit and vegetables. Although this will not harm you, the goal is to maximize the digestive process, and these two foods do not mix well in digestion. Fruits move quickly, from the stomach to the small intestine within 30 minutes, where they continue to digest. When eaten with vegetables and other foods that take several hours to enter the small intestine, the fruit is held up and starts to ferment, resulting in poor assimilation of nutrients and, more importantly, this creates a perfect environment for yeast cultures that feed off the sugar. Eat fruit and vegetables at least an hour and a quarter apart.

• Eat tomatoes. Though a fruit, they are okay with vegetables. They mix well.

• Alcohol: if you drink, limit yourself to one 2-ounce cocktail of hard liquor (vodka preferred), or one to two glasses of red wine daily. If one wishes to drink more than the recommended amounts, this regimen will still work, but it will not be as effective. It is important to remember that alcohol converts to sugar in our bodies: beer and white wine the most, and vodka the least.

• Treats: when you dine out, eat what is presented to you. Enjoy yourself! At home treat yourself on a periodic basis.

• Read nutritional information on the food packages you purchase. Remember "fat free" does not necessarily mean low-calorie, nor does it mean "sugarless" or "salt-free."

• Don't count calories. We should be calorie aware, but the real culprit is the fat gram. Calorie-counting complicates. It turns a simple plan into an arithmetic exercise. Calorie counting also opens the door to cheating: "I ate a banana split, but I really saved calories by skipping lunch." Remember, you must eat three meals a day. The goal is to achieve the Objectives of Nutrition, not simply lose weight.

• Switch to olive oil, extra-virgin cold press. It may seem expensive, but a little goes a long way. Olive oil contains the "good" cholesterol, but it is still a fat. Use it in moderation.

•Eliminate butter and margarine. Use olive oil on bread; use olive oil and a squeeze of lemon juice on vegetables.

• Change your meat eating habits. Adults do not need as much animal protein as recommended in the American food pyramid. Small portions of skinless chicken or turkey, or fish, combined with pasta, rice, legumes or any combination of vegetables will provide variety and excellent nutrition. Lean red meat should be eaten very sparingly.

• Eat more fruit and vegetables, at least one daily serving of cruciferous vegetables (broccoli, cabbage, cauliflower, mustard greens, turnips) and one daily serving of beta-carotene vegetables (carrots, kale, spinach, sweet potatoes). For fruits, eat apples, bananas, plums, apricots, cantaloupe, mangoes, nectarines, papayas, peaches, etc. Remember: do not combine fruits and vegetables, and try to eat a total of seven fruits and vegetables each day.

• Eat whole grain bread. Bake your own or find a bakery that produces country-style loaves with plenty of flavor. Most people think bread is fattening, but a slice of whole grain bread is no more fattening than an apple. Bread is primarily made from flour, water, yeast and salt. It is rich in complex carbohydrates, and a low-fat source of fiber, vitamins and minerals. Just be sure your bread is not made from refined flour.

Foods To Avoid

The following foods are to be avoided most times, and are only okay on a limited or occasional basis:

• Juices: use minimal fruit and vegetable juices. With extracted juices you miss most of the detoxifying and nourishing benefits of the whole fruit or vegetable, including disease-fighting phytochemicals. Most commercial juices simply extract the liquid from the fruit or vegetable, leaving behind cellulose and fiber, enzyme rich phytochemicals, and vitamins and minerals to nourish and heal the body. This process makes most juices out of balance foods and they lack the digestive aids of the fruit and vegetables from which they are extracted. Fruit juices in particular cause sharp and immediate increases in sugar levels in the body, and such increases are followed frequently by similarly quick drops in energy and alertness. Although we are not counting calories, fruit juices, including tomato juice, contain more calories than most people suspect. For nutritional benefits, whole fruits or vegetables are far superior.

• Non-Cultured Milk & Dairy Products: Quite simply, milk is an irritant to the system. Your body does require calcium and oil-soluble Vitamins A and D that are found in dairy products, particularly milk. The problem with these non-cultured dairy products is that they contain milk sugars that are hard on digestion, and maximizing digestion is one of the objectives of *21st Century Fitness* nutrition. Cultured dairy products such as kefir and yogurt are non-stressful to digestion, because the milk sugars have been converted to usable lactose and galactose by specialized "lactic acid" micro-organisms.

• Salt: use minimal amounts. Sodium intake appears to be linked to hypertension, an ailment that leads to heart attacks, strokes and kidney failure.

• Refined Sugar: the body needs sugar. Glucose, the main sugar in the blood and a basic fuel of the body, is essential to cell function—-especially those in the brain. However, we don't need to eat sugar to supply glucose. All we need is complex carbohydrates, or starches, which are found in foods derived from plants: grains, vegetables and fruits. Any eating regimen that does not include a substantial amount of glucose denies the body one of its most important foods. Many of the fad diets eliminate fruits and grains—the complex carbohydrates. I think this is a serious omission, because one of the key principles of *21st Century Fitness* nutrition is to obtain natural sugars from complex carbohydrates. In addition, refined sugar, as with fruit juices, creates a sharp increase in the sugar level in the body, and such increases are, again, followed frequently by similarly quick drops in energy and alertness, and cause mood swings. This works against another of the objectives of the *21st Century Fitness* nutritional plan. Finally, some of the latest studies indicate that the excessive consumption of refined sugars greatly increases the chances for myocardial infraction (heart attack) or diabetes.

• White Enriched (Refined) Flour: it lacks the bran and germ of the wheat grain, and there is less fiber. Most of the lost nutrition is not replaced, even in so-called "enriched" flour, which has only niacin, thiamin, riboflavin and iron added.

• Bagels: though they are virtually fat-free, most bagels contain between 300 and 400 calories. With butter, cream cheese, jelly, etc., bagels can be quite fattening. Furthermore, they are usually made from refined flour, and therefore the calories are "empty". If you must eat bagels, eat them sparingly.

• Prepared salad dressings: most are made from questionable ingredients and usually have significant amounts of fat. It is preferable to make your own from an olive oil and apple cider vinegar base.

• Mayonnaise: "Hold the mayo!" Regular mayonnaise is an emulsion of oil, egg yolk and vinegar—-and almost 100% fat.

• Ketchup: While it is made primarily from tomatoes, the average ketchup is 20% refined sugars and contains up to 180 milligrams of sodium per tablespoon. Even so called "lite" ketchup has a high sodium level.

• Red Meats: the problem with red meat can be summed up in two words: "fat" and "cholesterol."

• Fried Foods: too much fat for nutrition received. One of the key principles of *21st Century Fitness* nutrition is low fat intake.

• Bacon: tastes great, but look at the fat!

• Cereals: most packaged cereals are loaded with sugar, and in many cases, salt. Read labels.

• Peanut Butter: Most peanut butters are made with sugar additives, and the "naturals" are still loaded with fat grams: 16 in just two table-spoons, with 190 calories.

• Waffles, Pancakes, Rolls, Biscuits, Crackers: most are made from refined flour, which lacks the germ, and many contain sodium. One ounce of saltine crackers contain 130 calories and 3 grams of fat. But the biggest problem with these foods is what you put on them (syrup, butter, cheese, etc.) They almost always contain too much fat or sugar.

• Vegetable Oils: (except olive oil) —-all are merely fat in liquid form, and contain 120 calories and 13.5 grams of fat per tablespoon.

• Soft Drinks/Corn Syrup: while the use of refined sugar (sucrose) has dropped since 1975, the total amount of sugars in the American diet has remained the same. This is due to increased use of corn syrup, particularly the very sweet, high-fructose corn syrup now used in most sodas and many processed foods.

21st Century Fitness "Core" Foods

This is only a framework. It does not attempt to list every single accept-able food, just those that are readily available at most supermarkets.

Once you understand the principles you will find the other foods that work.

Dairy Foods

Yogurt (plain, fat-free)
Kefir

Vegetables

Lentils	Turnips
Broccoli	Cauliflower
Celery	Carrots
Beets	Parsley
Spinach	Watercress
Kale	Onions
Dark Leaf Lettuce	
Bok Choy	
Squash (all varieties)	
Sweet Potatoes (yams)	
Peas and Beans (all types)	
Hot Peppers (release endorphins, speed metabolism)	
Mushrooms (shitakes & portabellas are anti-cancer)	
Peppers (green, red & yellow)	

Fruits

Pomegranate	Kiwi
Apples (one per day)	Apricots
Oranges	Guavas
Grapefruit	Plums
Peaches	Cherries (limited amounts)
Watermelon	Dried Fruit (limited amounts)
Prunes (dried plums)	Bananas
Cantaloupe	Raisins
Honeydew	Blackberries
Tomatoes*	Blueberries
Lemons (one per day)	Tibetan Gogi Berries**
Grapes (limited amounts)	Elder Berries**
Nectarines	Choke Berries**
Tangerines	Cranberries** (1/2 c. dried or fresh daily)

Even though a fruit, tomatoes are a catalyst and should be used with vegetables.

**Highest level of antioxidants (much more than blueberries)*

Grains

Oats	Whole Grain Breads
Brown Rice	Grape Nuts (or generic)
Polenta	Pasta (made from whole grain flour)
Tabuleh	Couscous
Kasha	Barley
Bulgur	Kamut
Millet	Amaranth
Rye	Buckwheat
Corn	Triticale

ANTI - AGING AT ITS BEST

Meat & Fish

Cod	Skinless Turkey Breast
Salmon (wild only)	Skinless Chicken Breast
Haddock	Lean Red Meat (max. 4x a month)
Halibut	Sea Bass
Snapper	Swordfish
Trout	Shellfish (limited amounts)
Tuna (fresh)	Tuna (canned: water pack)

Assorted Foods

Tomato Sauce (organic: read labels for sugar and salt content)
Tofu
Garlic
Tabasco
Dry Spices
Dry Condiments, Herbs
Wheat Germ*
Apple Cider Vinegar
Flax Seeds
Raw Almonds (no more than 12 a day) (refrigerate)
Olive Oil (extra virgin, cold press) (keep in dark place or refrigerate)
Oregano (use often)
Honey (raw, unheated)
Pickles (limited amounts)
Mustard (any kind, dry preferred)

* Two tablespoons of wheat germ contain
   more protein than 1/4 lb. of hamburger

Beverages

Teas (herbal)
Coffee (minimal, caffeine acceptable)
Green tea (One of the most powerful antioxidants)

Mange, Mange! Enjoy!

The list of "core" foods in *21st Century Fitness* nutrition is designed to stimulate the imagination to the variety of flavors, textures, aromas, and colors of the dishes you design for yourself. You are encouraged to experiment! The list is by no means complete. There are literally hundreds of specialty foods, ethnic foods, varieties of fruits, grains and vegetables, even meats that are native to isolated regions of the world. The only cautionary advice is to check the type of food you are buying to be sure it falls within the general nutritional plan outlined.

In these times of two or more people in a household working outside the home, convenience plays a role in your food selection and preparation. Refrigerator containers for certain basic "old reliables" that are already pre-pared will save time. They are excellent for storing pre-prepared brown rice, beans, pasta, couscous, tabuleh, etc. With these you can "build" a meal to your preference at any time and very quickly.

A Daily Regimen

The significant principle of a daily regimen is to eliminate fringe foods and to eat large quantities of the right foods. It is important to eat three meals a day, and snacks three times a day to maximize metabolism and to never feel hungry. Missing meals slows down the metabolism, resulting in weight gain, mood swings and loss of energy. The elimination of a meal or snack throws everything out of balance. The idea is to achieve the Objectives of Nutrition.

Immediately upon rising, drink one cup of hot water with 1/2 to a whole lemon squeezed into it.

Breakfast:

(At least 20 minutes after hot water with lemon).
1 or 2 cups of caffeinated coffee is okay.

During the day, drink at least eight 8-ounce glasses of water.

Mid-morning, one apple.

Lunch:

Mid-afternoon, one fruit of your choice and 12 raw almonds.

Dinner:

Evening - anytime an hour and a quarter after dinner —
if you have a craving for sweets, eat 2 or 3
21st Century Fitness cookies.*
(Fat-free, sugarless and made from whole grain flour)

Late night, before retiring, eat one whole Grapefruit.
(Or 1/2 if a whole is too much.)

* *21st Century Fitness* cookies can be ordered from *21st Century* Enterprises.

ANTI - AGING AT ITS BEST

Here are some examples and suggestions for your meals:

Breakfast: To grape nuts or hot oat bran add as much as you want of fruit and non-fat yogurt and one tablespoon of wheat germ, one tablespoon of honey (raw unheated) and one tablespoon of flax seed oil. Mix well. There are other breakfasts, such as fruit alone, and they fall into the utility meal category—-fast, tasty, energizing-that enable us to get on with the day.

Skip breakfast, gain weight! According to Dr. Isadore Rosenfeld, many studies have shown that omitting breakfast actually adds pounds. Here's why: After fasting all night, you're likely to have hunger pangs long before lunch. The snack you take-some potato chips or cookies-is likely to contain plenty of calories, salt, sugar and fat. But psychologically you think that's OK, because you didn't have breakfast. Skipping breakfast will increase your weight by another mechanism too. Your body reacts as if there's no food available. It wants to protect you against starvation. So when you finally do eat, you don't burn the calories-you hang on to them and store them as fat to be used when the "famine" has ended. Stored fat means extra pounds. By contrast, the high fiber and low fat in cereals can prevent weight gain or even induce weight loss. Eating at least 21 grams of soluble fiber a day (other things being equal) can leave you pounds lighter.

Lunch: Whether salad, soup, sandwich or traditional divided meal, combine and mix from the universe of suggested foods. Whole grain carbohydrates such as bread or pasta should be eaten at this meal only. They will be used as energy for the rest of the day. You simply must include large portions of vegetables. Remember: no fruit at lunch; eat with breakfast & between meals.

Dinner: An example: heat a skillet with olive oil, add garlic, onions, tomatoes, and your cruciferous and beta carotene vegetables. If you are not having turkey, chicken or fish, beans are a must; They provide the protein you need. While the foods are cooking, have a glass of iced tea or a vodka martini. This recipe can also be made as a casserole. If you prefer, add an egg to bind the ingredients. (Eggs are acceptable, but no more than 2-3 per week.) Be sure to add a carrot or two which will act as a natural sweetener.

You may prefer a meal that is neatly divided: a breast of chicken, your beans, your vegetables, salad—-all served individually in a more traditional manner. Use the list of "core" foods and your imagination! The important thing to remember is that you are not on a diet. You are eating the right foods for nutrition and enjoyment. Be patient. Give this plan a chance to work.

A Rule Of Thumb

A rule of thumb to gauge the intake of carbohydrates, fat and protein is the following: 70% of the daily calories required by the body should come from carbohydrates (fruits, vegetables, and whole grains), 10% from fats (olive oil, flax seed, soy and nuts), and 20% from proteins (fish, fowl, wheat germ and legumes).

Weight Control

21st Century Fitness offers a nutrition plan. It is not a diet. For those who want and need to lose weight, this nutrition plan, unlike a diet, is a method to lose weight permanently. Statistics show that most diets work for weight reduction initially, but most people regain the weight, and frequently more weight than when they started as a result of their altered metabolisms.

21st Century Fitness nutrition fulfills the Objectives of Nutrition and stabilizes weight for those who do not have a weight problem. They will not lose weight. A person that is too thin will gain weight to an optimum level. An overweight person will lose weight until reaching their optimum weight level.

Finally, the idea is that achieving the right weight is a slow process, a natural adjustment for the metabolism. And that is the secret of its success.

It is important to eat three meals a day and snacks three times a day to maximize metabolism and to never feel hungry. Missing meals slows down the metabolism, resulting in weight gain, mood swings, and loss of energy. The elimination of a meal or snack throws everything out of balance. The idea is to achieve the **Objectives of Nutrition.**

Vitamins, Minerals & Supplements

Vitamins are organic substances that the body requires to help regulate metabolic functions. They are absolutely essential to life. Among the myriad of tasks they perform are:

- **Promoting good vision**
- **Forming normal blood cells**
- **Creating strong bones and teeth**
- **Ensuring the proper function of the heart and nervous system**

Researchers have uncovered the role vitamins play in preventing the damaging effects of oxygen on essential chemicals in the body. While vitamins themselves do not supply energy, some do aid in the efficient conversion of foods into energy. In general, vitamins must be consumed because our bodies cannot manufacture them. Until recently, medical authorities have been reluctant to recommend vitamins on a broad scale for healthy people eating healthy diets. However, the accumulation of research in recent years has prompted a change in attitude, at least in regard to four specific vitamins. These are the so-called antioxidant vitamins, plus the B vitamin, folacin. The role these substances play in disease prevention is no longer a matter of dispute.

Ideally your vitamins should come from your diet rather than from pills. Indeed, supplements cannot substitute for a healthy diet, but even if you do eat very well, and most Americans do not, it is unlikely you will get the high levels of folacin and of the antioxidant vitamins many authorities think you need.

Scientists have been paying great attention to minerals in recent years, looking for links between them and the major chronic diseases: high blood pressure, osteoporosis, cardio-vascular disease, diabetes and even cancer. The minerals that are nutrients are absolutely essential to a host of vital processes in the body, from the basic bone formation and enzyme synthesis to the regulation of the heart muscle and the normal functioning of digestion. Many are necessary for the activity of enzymes, proteins that serve as catalysts in the body's chemical reactions. Unlike the organic compounds we call vitamins, minerals are inorganic substances, that is, they do not contain carbon. Carried into the soil, ground water, and sea by erosion, they are taken up by plants and consumed by plants and humans. Minerals in food are indestructible; even if you burn your food to a cinder, it will retain all its original minerals. *But over-boiling food can deplete food of mineral content.*

It is preferable to see a medically-trained doctor of nutrition who can prescribe a nutrition supplement after a complete blood analysis. This is what Dr. Cott did for me. In lieu of a medically-trained doctor or qualified alternative medicine practitioner who might prescribe a far more personalized and complex supplement plan, the following list is a recommendation of universal benefit:

One of the following per day, taken with one of your meals:

One multi vitamin with minerals, plus...		
Vitamin C	1000 mg.	Antioxidant; cold prevention; cancer
Vitamin E	400 I. U.	Antioxidant
Vitamin B Complex	100 mg.	Helps in formation of red blood cells
Selenium	100 mg.	Antioxidant to fight cell damage
Niacin	250 mg.	Converts carbohydrates to energy, produces red blood cells
Zinc	50 mg.	Immune system, cell growth and repair
CoQ10	(Gel Form)	Antioxidant
Magnesium	50 mg.	Energy production, reproduction, building bones
Melatonin		Optional
Calcium Citrate	250 mg.	Bone density and strength, teeth, helps prevent osteoporosis
B-12	100 mg.	Necessary for development of red blood cells
Folic Acid	250 mg.	Antioxidant
Flax Seed Oil		Follow dosage recommended
Spirulina		Take as directed.

Vitamin and mineral supplements alone have very little value, however, combined with proper nutrition their value is substantial.

The Completed Picture

This chapter on nutrition completes the formula for *21st Century Fitness*. As the Empire State Building was built floor by floor, we have built this formula step by step. And as the critical elements in construction are design and materials, the critical elements in this formula are exercise and nutrition. As the architect's goal is to raise up a building that will endure, the goal of *21st Century Fitness*. is to provide a formula for the human body to retain or regain its youth. The formula is complete. Now it is yours.

Without proper nutrition you cannot achieve all *8 Essentials of Fitness*. Nutrition is not isolated as exercise should not be isolated. The two are mutually codependent in building fitness

My *21st Century Fitness* Students

It is no coincidence that the majority of my students come to me dissatisfied and frustrated in regards to their attempts to achieve fitness. Most are products of state of the art gyms and certified personal trainers, yet no matter how hard they've worked they feel something has been missing. And they're right. What's been missing is a specific formula of fitness and nutrition that will give them all *8 Essentials of Fitness* and allow them to become *8 Essential Fit*. Instead, they've followed methods that have only allowed them to be partially fit. Fortunately, they've discovered the **21st Century Fitness** formula.

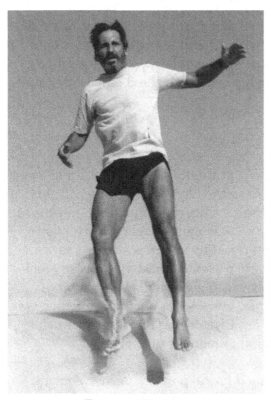

Ramon Duncan

Ramon Duncan, 53

I'm 53 years old, and given my strong, muscular physique, I've been thought by many to be in remarkable shape, especially for my age. Sure, with intense free weight training I had the appearance of fitness; I even had a five miles a day running regimen that assured people (and myself) that I was in the best of shape. It wasn't until I began training with Larry that I realized how limited my body actually was and how hard I'd been working to remain unfit.

But at first I was skeptical. I knew Larry casually, and though it was obvious that he had employed an extraordinarily effective method of exercise — knowing his age, he was truly amazing. But how could his method possibly yield better results than my 5 mile a day run, and three days a week in the gym? How could he say I was unfit? My curiosity was peeked and my ego challenged. At his invitation, I came to his house to see just what it was he was talking about, and as he began to workout on the mat I thought to myself, "you've got to be kidding, this is a piece of cake." Then I tried the workout myself. I was astonished. Here I was, so sure and proud of my physical abilities, and I was so tight and inflexible I could barely get through the warm up. I was straining and puffing, groaning and perspiring. Finally I was able to make it through merely six of the exercises. It was then that I reevaluated my concept of what it meant to be fit.

I continued to train with Larry. Within two months I was noticing my already muscular body awakening to a level of fitness far beyond what I could have ever imagined. I learned that much of my weight training had been counterproductive because it had tightened and over-built my muscles, reinforcing imperfections in my body's structure. I came to realize that only certain weight training exercises, and then only when they're done in the right amounts, are really effective. They serve as enrichment to the floor work and fill-ins, the foundation of Larry's formula. It's not about quantity, either. Why should it matter how much you can lift if you are unable to touch your toes?

Today, I still go to the gym to do the weight portions of the formula, but I find it upsetting when I see how many people are being blindly led down paths with conventional ideas of fitness. It's frustrating, too, because I understand that they believe what they're doing will provide them with all they need—-I was one of them!—I just wish I could make them realize no matter how hard you workout, no matter what results you may see, if you don't have a complete formula that provides you with the 8 essentials, you're selling yourself short.

Allison Temple, M. D., 40

I'm 40, and until five years ago, I had continually searched for an effective and appropriate exercise regimen since the days of my residency. I tried jogging, and I joined health club after health club, working out on machines with young, muscled trainers. Like many, I was vainly trying to trim down, but in my efforts I began to notice a deterioration in my posture. I saw my future in my elderly rigid and osteoporotic patients, and I was already feeling that future in my neck and back. I began to experience quite a bit of pain. Some of it was brought on by stress, but a large part of my aching was a direct result from exercises and training I was doing at the gym, much of which only reinforced the curve and nonalignment of my spine.

Despite my medical training, I searched for help in the women's magazines I read on the Stairmaster. It was in one of these magazines that I learned of Pilates. The theories behind it made sense, so I found a studio that offered this "new" method of training. Much to my disappointment my progress was slow and minimal, and nothing was being done to increase my flexibility or correct my posture, let alone to alleviate my pain. As I found out later, there are many studios that teach Pilates, but unless the instructors have been trained or certified by someone from the original New York studio, you might receive a "whisper down the lane" version of Pilates' training. That is exactly what happened to me.

I was still searching for a truly effective method of exercise when I happened to meet Larry Nachman at a party given by my mother. We spoke for quite a while, and he left me with the impression of a very fit, youthful man somewhere in his mid 40s. It came as a great shock when I found out he was 65. As a doctor, I'm usually very good at determining someone's age, and I became excited and intrigued that someone could be his age and have not only a lean, well proportioned body, but also have such a free range of motion and a high level of energy. When I found out that he was a trainer, it really got my attention. He had exactly what I always wanted: to be young in my later years. Immediately it crossed my mind that if I did what he did I would probably get similar results. Later that week I started my training with Larry.

It took a little bit of time to get used to the routine, but after only seven months of mat work, my back was straighter, more supple and virtually pain-free. My whole body was toned and looked more youthful. What's more, I wasn't spending hours and hours at the gym, and given my busy schedule, this is especially worth noting. Now, after two years of training with Larry, I'm in better condition than I could have ever expected. My neck is now straight and aligned; my posture is no longer flawed. Despite becoming fit to a degree that I didn't know existed, Larry tells me that I will only continue to improve.

Andrea Ziff Cooper, 35

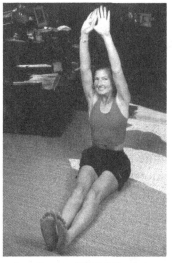

Andrea Ziff Cooper

I was only 26 when I started working out with Larry. Though he pointed out that I was one of the fortunate few who, in addition to being slim and well toned, also had naturally excellent posture, he also said there is always room for improvement. While Larry told me the changes I would see would not be drastic, he did say that my body would become more defined, my shoulders would become more square, and that I would notice improvements in my posture and flexibility. However, the most significant benefit he told me I would receive from his formula was that by achieving the *8 Essentials of Fitness* now, I would avoid going through the traditional aging process.

Larry was right. Eight months after I began my training I got married. When I tried on my wedding gown I was excited about the changes in my shoulders. As expected, I had noticed improved flexibility, but to see how much taller I was standing, how my posture had improved, made me think again about what Larry had said about the aging process. It's the most exciting aspect of Larry's formula.

I'd never thought about fitness as staying young. The idea never occurred to me. The fact is, I'd never given much thought to aging at all. I assumed that as long as I exercised I would be fit, but now I know there's a lot more to it.

Chuck Jennings, 43

It was March of '98, and I was 35. I was struggling through yet another workout at the Wellness Center of the Medical University of South Carolina, where it's said, "If you don't get fit here, you won't get fit anywhere." The Wellness Center was not my first attempt at getting fit. Since college I had tried everything I knew of and worked at each one diligently: weight training, circuit training, jogging, assorted aerobic classes, yoga, kick-boxing, Tai Chi, Stairmasters, stationary bikes, rowing machines, treadmills...you get the picture? It's hard to describe my frustration caused by exercising hard and dieting rigorously to end up with a body that's misshapen—-head pitched forward, curved spine, sloped shoulders, caved-in chest, wide hips and flared thighs. Even though my muscles had become more toned, my structure was still flawed. I suppose, yes, I had become fitter, but the proportions remained. As I honed in on middle age I was becoming convinced that I was doomed to be a genetic pear.

Huffing and puffing, dripping wet, I happened to look across the room and noticed a man talking to one of the personal trainers. What got my attention was that I could tell he was somewhat older than the trainer, and yet he looked much fitter. It was a different kind of fitness, though. He had the body of a young athlete—-sleek, stretched and muscular without bulk, but what struck me the most was his high chest and straight shoulders. Suddenly it dawned on me that in all the years of trying to get fit, I never knew exactly what I wanted, but finally there it was. For the first time I was seeing it. Up until then the trainers I had worked under were my models, but I suddenly realized it wasn't their muscular bulk that I wanted, but that long, lean look like the man across the room.

Thirty minutes later, having reinforced my gloom by looking in the mirror, I came out of the showers and three lockers from mine was this man with a different kind of fitness. Larry introduced himself, and I began talking. I told him how hard I'd worked to get such poor results, and I asked him what he did. He told me he followed a formula that he had developed over the years, that it was quick, easy, and that it filled in the links missing in conventional fitness programs. He went on to explain that the foundation for the formula was a floorwork routine that reshaped and realigned the body. I was surprised to discover he was a trainer, and I was impressed enough to schedule a workout.

But after two months I had my doubts. I was showing progress, but nothing much more than I had achieved in the past. I could always lose weight, so the only difference was that I seemed to be more flexible, and I was feeling muscles that I had never felt before. However, changes were not happening fast enough. I was getting tempted to do more, and everyone was suggesting something better.

In the past I had succumbed to that temptation to do more and more, but without success. This time, for some reason, I kept listening to Larry. He told me I didn't need more, that I didn't need anything else, that all I needed was to simply follow the formula. "Do it over and over and over, again and again and again. Don't waver. You will get the *8 Essentials of Fitness*." I did it over and over, again and again. I did not waver, and in twelve months my waist went from a 39 plus to 31 inches. My "genetic" hips and thighs literally melted away. My shoulders grew high, my caved chest became full, and my neck straightened. Physically, I became everything I wanted to be, and it was because of this exact exercise regimen and nutritional plan. Weight loss and a conventional exercise regimen would never have come close to giving me what I have today. It never did.

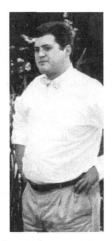   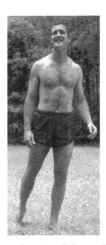

Chuck Jennings, March 1998   Chuck Jennings, March 1999

Melanie McLamb, 42

I'm 42, and I started working out with Larry when I was 34. He was the fitness "guru" retained as trainer by Ziff Properties in Charleston, South Carolina, the company where I worked. At the time, years of horseback riding, work outs at the gym and sensible eating habits kept me trim. Cosmetically I was satisfied with my appearance and thought I was physically fit.

I was in for a surprise.

From the start I believed Larry's formula would work for me. I loved the idea that it was fast, as I did it in my lunch hour and still had time for lunch. But I had no idea that the benefits of *21st Century Fitness* would be so much more than just keeping me "fit." I learned there was a level of fitness I didn't know about. The results were beyond my wildest expectations.

Today I'm complimented on my perfect posture, and I'm lean and toned in a way that I could not have imagined. I have tremendous strength and far more flexibility than I had even as an accomplished equestrian. My energy level is wonderful. But the biggest surprise is that now I'm instructing others in the ways of **21st Century Fitness**. So many have asked me how I achieved my noteworthy physical condition that I decided to help spread Larry's message. I can now open people's eyes to a new way of life just as Larry did for me.

Ella Richardson, 40+

I almost gave up on **21st Century Fitness** because I kept thinking that surely I wasn't doing enough, that I needed to perspire more, to work harder. Larry assured me that all I needed was to stick to the formula, and fortunately I listened. With practice and patience I realized that Larry was right, that less was indeed more, and my entire outlook on fitness has changed.

Jeannie Cerni, 80+

In 1945 I was a student of Joseph Pilates at his original studio in New York. As a ballet dancer I have an understanding of the body, and I knew

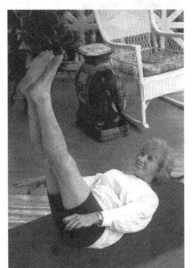

Jeannie Cerni

that his method of exercise was vital to keeping myself in prime physical condition, although many of my friends thought we Pilates' students were kooks. And no wonder! I remember climbing those spooky stairs, the strange looking machines, and Joseph's wife, Clara, in her nurse's uniform. Those workouts, though, were just wonderful.

In those days, Pilates referred to what we now call the mat work as "contrology." Contrology consisted of 34 movements on the mat, the core of the Pilates method. Joe was pictured doing the mat exercises at age 60 and was the epitome of long-lasting youth. Larry has taken 21 of those core exercises to make up the foundation of the **21st Century Fitness** formula. I enjoy training with him not only because it's quick and complete, but to see the youth Larry exhibits inspires and exhilarates me. It's a quality of fitness I remember in my old trainer Joe (only better).

ANTI - AGING AT ITS BEST

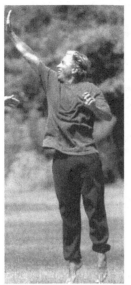

Scott Settle

Scott Settle, 58

When I was in my 20s I worked out avidly. I had been an all-round athlete in college, but as I grew older I didn't think I'd ever experience that feeling of supreme fitness again. Today, however, I'm 58 and in better shape, more fit, than I was at 25, and it's because of the *21st Century Fitness* formula.

Before I started with Larry I was working out six days a week: bicycling, walking, stair-stepping, rowing, and circuit training. I was far from unfit. In fact for someone over 50 I was in great shape. I felt great, and I thought I had pretty good flexibility. What more did I need? It was my wife who talked me into going to one of Larry's classes, and at first I didn't really want to go. But when I saw him I realized he possessed a level of fitness I thought was impossible to achieve at my age, let alone over 60. I suddenly knew that I could re-experience the fitness of my youth, for that's exactly what Larry had—-the fitness of a man in his 20s.

My first experience with the floor work confirmed my initial judgment, and I began using muscles and stretching in ways I had never experienced before. After the first workout Larry explained to me his *8 Essentials of Fitness*, and for the first time the specifics of what I sought became clear. Right then I committed myself to following the *21st Century Fitness* formula—-everything, including the nutrition.

By the fourth month it all started to come together. The man is right on! I must say that up until then, although I never once doubted the end results, there were things that I questioned. At that point however, when I finally began to see and feel results far beyond what I'd so recently thought impossible, I realized there was no need to question. It's the precision and efficiency of the formula that works.

Carole Settle, 50+

It sounds dramatic, but it's true, so I'm comfortable saying it: Larry Nachman's *21st Century Fitness* formula has been a life-changing experience for me. I have so much more energy, and I've never felt stronger or fitter, especially in my back and abs, which for a potter like myself is cause for celebration. My entire disposition has changed because the way I look is in complete agreement with the way I feel. I've lost 15 pounds, and with my new muscle tone I'm able to wear styles and sizes of clothes that were a fantasy before.

ANTI - AGING AT ITS BEST

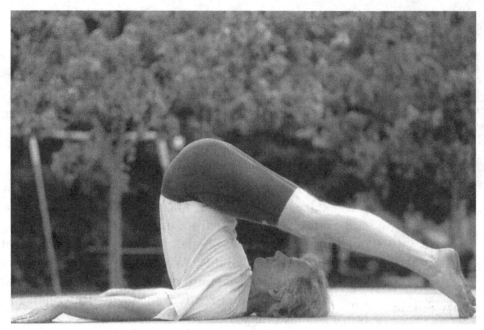

Lyle Allen

Lyle Allen, 55

I was a student of Yoga for many years, and over time I became an instructor. Gradually, my ability to perform complicated stretches increased my strength and flexibility to a point where I believed I was in exceptional condition, and to a certain extent I was. My wife, however, had begun searching for a more effective exercise program. More effective than Yoga? How could that be possible?

Soon she said she'd found an exercise class that called for her to use her body and muscles in a new way. Her enthusiasm for the methods taught in her new class, and her claims that they might be better than Yoga, piqued my curiosity. I had to see for myself. While watching one of my wife's classes I became intrigued with what I began to realize was a specific formula. It appeared that maybe my wife was right, and soon I joined her in her classes with Larry.

The first thing I discovered was the weakness of what Larry termed my "powerhouse." I thought my stomach muscles were well developed, but Larry showed me how much stronger they could be. As the months progressed I found myself more and more committed to his formula, and I particularly enjoyed seeing the result of using dumbbells.

Given my long association with Yoga, I was aware of the important benefits of deep stretching, but now I was realizing it was ***stretching coupled***

with resistance that made the difference in building supple strength. When combined with a nutritional plan built on common sense, I realized I was in possession of an extremely well balanced regimen. Within another month or two my body had strengthened and realigned to a point where my posture improved significantly. Now I realize that while certainly there are benefits that come from practicing Yoga, alone it fails to provide a complete and balanced formula like *21st Century Fitness*.

Patty Granthem, 49

Even at 47, when I started with Larry, I never understood that posture and alignment of the body were the core elements of staying young. Today I can't help but have a profound understanding of this truth since my body continues to stretch and get taller with every workout.

Laura Beckstrom, 70+

At 67 I never thought I'd be able to do a sit-up with my hands clasped behind my head, but Larry kept telling me to be patient and it would happen. It took five months, but he was right. Now my body has strength I thought was impossible for someone my age to attain. Furthermore, because Larry's formula requires virtually no equipment, I find that my frequent traveling doesn't impede my workout schedule at all. One might say that I'm a portable gym.

Suzanne Seymour, 70+

I love my chocolates! And I've chosen not to give them up, so I'm not one of Larry's students who follows the nutritional plan of *21st Century Fitness*. The exercises, however, are another matter. They are an imperative part of my life, and they've allowed me to maintain a dynamic schedule without the limitations I was beginning to experience before I met Larry.

At 66 I was getting "old" - weak, inflexible, low energy - and this was not acceptable. I was very aware I needed something, but I wasn't quite sure what it would be. In 1997 I was attending a water aerobics class at the Family "Y" and saw Larry showing a very physically fit woman what looked to me to be a strange exercise. I inquired and he told me it was part of his floor work routine in a formula he had developed to attain youth in his later years. To see Larry's tone and flexibility was proof enough for me. I went to work with Larry's formula, and refused to let my age prevent me from learning the exercises. It took some time, but eventually I was able to perform all of the floor work and fill-ins. I'm now past 70, yet I find I have as much flexibility, strength and energy as ever. The exercises in *21st Century Fitness* have allowed me to recapture my youth, and I still eat my chocolates.

Beth Nachman Riley, 44

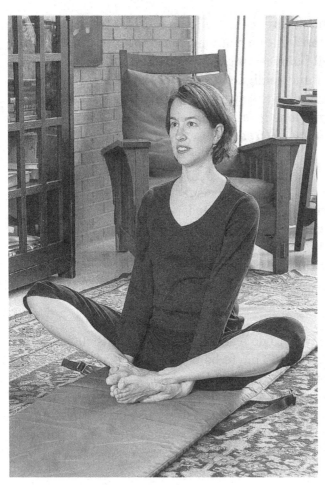

Beth Nachman Riley

When I was 14 I would look forward to attending Saturday morning sessions with my father and brother at the Pilates studio in New York. I continued to do my mat work intermittently over the years, and in 1998 I began to follow my dad's ***21st Century Fitness*** formula. When I became pregnant with my first child at age 36, I continued with the floor work. After the fifth month I eliminated the exercises that called for lying on my stomach, but I used all the other elements of the formula until six weeks before the baby was born. Amazingly, not only did I feel great, but I looked great, too! There was nothing different about my body other than the enlarged stomach. The usual bloated arms and legs never materialized.

Six weeks after the birth of my baby I resumed the program. As you might imagine, trying to schedule a workout while getting used to being a mother was not exactly easy, but given the efficiency and effectiveness of the ***21st Century Fitness*** formula, within another eight weeks my body was better than ever. In this case the old adage rings true: father does know best.

Bob Nachman, 42

I was the epitome of the saying "All That Glitters Is Not Gold." At 37 I thought I basically had the same physical qualities I did when I was on my Prep School swim team. My workouts consisted of free weight training and 2 miles a day in the pool, but as I crossed the threshold of what my father calls the "cross-over age," I began to feel my body's limitations. When I evaluated myself in the mirror I thought I looked physically fit, yet I found I couldn't touch my toes. I was flexibly impaired.

Even though it was hard to let go of my conventional ideas about staying in shape, I finally surrendered, and asked my father to show me the floor work and fill-in exercises that make up his **21st Century Fitness** formula. Now I am totally flexible and have all *8 Essentials of Fitness*. I'm in better condition than when I was on my prep school swim team.

Sally Youngblood, 62

In August of 2001, I was a 57 year old runner who was gaining weight and stiffening more each year.

That spring, I ruptured a disc and had other injuries, resulting from heavy gardening and house renovating.

I started doing the **21st Century Fitness** formula with Larry Nachman on August 15, 2001. I liked it so much that one month later I followed his advice to walk instead of run. As time went on, I began to feel stronger in my back. First the aches and pains went away. Then I began to notice I was slimmer and, very noticeably, more flexible.

On January 15, 2002, I had a single mastectomy on my left side and a modified mastectomy on my right side with an auxiliary node to levels I and II. I had Jackson-Pratt drains in both sides. I was told not to raise my arms above my shoulders for one week. Then I was told I could start creeping my hands up the wall. This seemed to do little for my general well being, so I began to do my **21st Century Fitness** floor work. I was unable to do any of the exercises on my stomach, but found the routine lying on my back helped combat the tightening feeling I was experiencing and made me feel much better. The drains worked themselves out and were removed.

I bought a softer mat and added the exercises back that were on my stomach. During this time I experienced more pain as my nerves were growing back, but I could tell things were improving. Three weeks after the operation, I was doing the entire routine, but my right arm was still tight as a result of the node dissection. After only one more week, one month after the operation, to my amazement and others I know who have had similar procedures, I was almost as stretched and strong as before the operation. My husband, who is a doctor, and I are convinced the floor work and fill-in exercises of **21st Century Fitness** was my way to a speedy and happy recovery. I've continued to get slimmer every day. My hips and stomach are melting away and all *8 Essentials of Fitness* that Larry speaks of is becoming reality. I'm at a level of fitness I never thought possible at my age!

ANTI - AGING AT ITS BEST

Lee Strickland, 44

Beyond my wildest dreams!

I am a golfer who I thought had incurable middle age spread. In 6 weeks of following the ***21st Century Fitness*** formula, I've lost 4 1/2 inches in my waist. I'm not hungry. I feel great and look great. I'm more flexible and to my surprise, my golf game has gotten better.

It's impossible to describe the joy I'm experiencing.

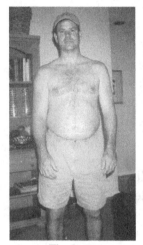 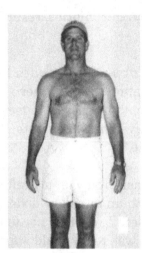 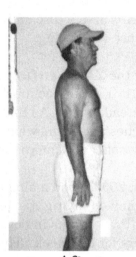 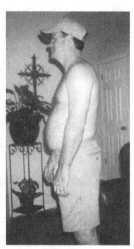

Before   *After*   *After*   *Before*

RESULTS IN JUST SIX WEEKS!

Our New Way of Thinking

As a group, we now understand that it takes a specific formula of exercise and nutrition to achieve our goals of fitness, whereas before our notion of fitness was only vague. We didn't have a clear vision of what we wanted. Our ideas of fitness simply revolved around the notion of "working out," but the qualities of fitness are defined by specific standards, just like when buying a diamond. As students we learned to question, "what fitness?" "Cardio-vascular fit?" "Muscularly fit?" "Flexibly fit?" "To what specific results? "At what age?" Most importantly we learned to look for proof that the program we follow provides all *8 Essentials of Fitness* like we found in Larry's formula, and as he says, "Don't pay the price for a fine diamond and end up with a flawed stone."

21st Century Fitness For All Ages

At the time of writing this book, I have 70 *21st Century Fitness* students: 42 women and 28 men. The age breakdown is as follows:

> **2 between 10 - 20**
> **4 between 20 - 30**
> **17 between 30 - 40**
> **9 between 40 - 50**
> **13 between 50 - 60**
> **20 between 60 - 70**
> **5 between 70 - 80**

Over the years, I've trained a number of students who learned the formula and now workout on their own, which is the one of the most significant advantages of the formula. And as you can tell from the range of ages, this formula is for everyone.

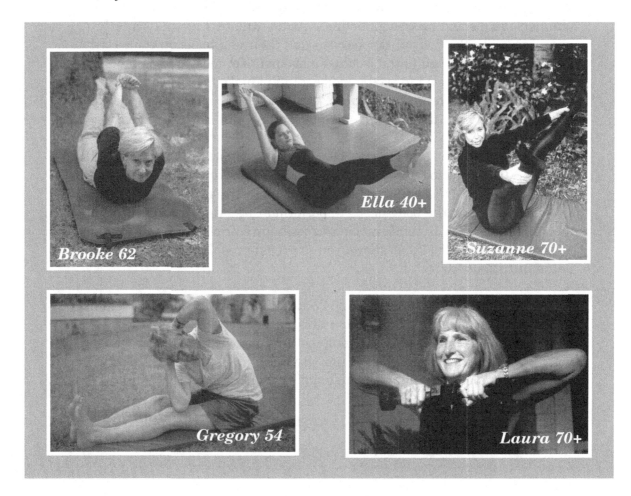

ANTI - AGING AT ITS BEST

Professional Opinions

As a physician, I've been inundated with fitness books, solicitations from gyms, and brochures for seminars that promise instant results to their subscribers and my patients. Although many of these programs offer sound guidance, I'm continually disappointed by the approach and methods usually outlined in their proposed attempts to achieve their stated goals. Often the advice and fitness programs are unnecessarily complicated, and too often they inspire unrealistic expectations. None that I can think of offer a complete and balanced formula.

I first met Larry at a social gathering and was astonished when he revealed his age. I thought he was a much younger man. In fact, I perceived him to be the most physically fit individual at the gathering, not simply the fittest person for his age. My curiosity was so roused that I had to find out what he did to maintain such a vibrant, youthful demeanor. In conversation Larry told me about his approach to fitness, and since then I've had an opportunity to read an early draft of this book.

What most intrigues me about Larry's methods to reclaim fitness are his uniquely simple and precise guidelines. As an athlete, I am particularly impressed with the floor work exercises and their emphasis on connected movements, as opposed to the isolated movements of most fitness programs. Larry has effectively addressed a modern individual's lifestyle by designing a formula that is simple and efficient, yet focused on combining proper diet, fluid movement and flexibility, resistance training and aerobic exercise.

I'm also impressed with Larry's common sense approach to eating. While it doesn't take a doctor to realize that exercise and nutrition go hand in hand, to maximize the effects of this pairing, however, it does take proper knowledge of what the body needs to perform at its best. Instead of recommending diet cycles or cumbersome recipes and restrictions, Larry provides a "lifetime grocery list" that allows you to prepare meals from a virtual arsenal of nutritious foods.

I believe this book will redefine the concept of fitness. It offers a complete and specific formula focused on the individual who seeks the eight essentials that will provide him or her with long lasting youth. Larry's message is a voice of empowerment, and it's simple. By following the *21st Century Fitness* formula you will be able to enjoy your later years to the fullest.

Bill Schmidt, M. D.
Charleston, South Carolina

As a physical therapist, I've compared Larry's approach to exercise to what I was taught in school and what I've seen in practice. There are many simi-

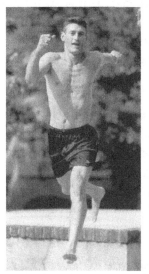

larities, but most significant are his focus on strength matched with flexibility, an emphasis on the abdomen and trunk, and the connection between mind and body, which is the most important concept in physical rehabilitation.

One of our shortcomings in physical therapy is that we focus on strengthening the affected muscle or joint and sometimes forget the whole person. The connected exercises that make up the floor work of *21st Century Fitness* are the biggest difference I see between Larry's formula and most strength building exercises. Each of his exercises incorporates a large number of muscle groups from head to toe. In addition to strength and flexibility, many of these movements help to improve balance and control. I find this combination of floor work, fill-ins, extra abdominal exercises and walking to

Bruce Reeves P.T.

be especially intriguing. Finally, the emphasis on the alignment of the spine and its ultimate effect on the structure of the body is what sets this formula apart from the majority of fitness regimens. I'm able to make these claims not just from reading a rough draft of this book, but because I was able to witness its effectiveness first hand.

In March of 1999, Chuck had sloped shoulders, a curved spine, flared hips, a pitched neck and was 50 pounds overweight. Along with those problems he was uncoordinated and struggled through his workouts at the Wellness Center at the Medical University of South Carolina. In March of 1999 Chuck was trim, had straight shoulders, a straight spine and a straight neck. He was a coordinated man whisking through his workouts. Watching Chuck's body change so dramatically in so short a time was amazing.

During this time we often would work out at the same time, so I would see him two or three times a week. Both of us were quite diligent in our training, and since we're roughly the same age, I could identify with his efforts. I also was aware of his poor posture, and as a physical therapist I would sometimes offer him suggestions as he moved from machine to machine. One day I noticed Chuck had made a complete turnabout. He was on the floor doing what looked like some yoga-style movement, but different. After that he moved to the dumbbells. All of this was done very quickly and then he was gone. He hadn't done his usual circuit training at all, and usually we were in the gym for about the same length of time. Something had happened.

When I talked to Chuck he told me he'd met Larry Nachman and was following his **21st Century Fitness** formula. I wished him well and didn't think any more about it. A few months later I saw Chuck perform a standing flip on the gym floor. I was astonished. Whatever Chuck had been doing with Larry's program was certainly working. He could have never done that before, and for the rest of the year I watched as Chuck's body was transformed.

I've seen people lose lots of weight, develop muscles and movement skills, but to see structural change is something else. To straighten a spine, a protruding neck and head, and to straighten shoulders is a rare accomplishment. In addition, I've had years of experience working out in gyms with certified trainers, and to know that Chuck was able to go so far as to correct his structure with Larry's formula has certainly broadened my thinking about fitness. There is no other method that I know of that could have generated the same results so quickly, if at all.

Bruce Reeves, P. T.
Charleston, South Carolina

Being a medical doctor specializing in reconstructive surgery, I am especially attuned to the physical appearance and anatomy of the body. It is also because of my specialty that I was so particularly fascinated by the transformation of Allison Temple, with whom I've worked closely over the last couple of years.

When I first met Allison I remember thinking that she was attractive, and on the surface she appeared to be a physically "together" young woman. But as I continued to see her on a more regular basis, I noticed that she had a curvature of the spine and that her head strained forward. I was aware that she worked out regularly, so I wasn't surprised when she mentioned that she was beginning a new fitness program. However as time went on, I began to notice a significant transformation in Allison's posture. I had since learned that her new program was something called **21st Century Fitness**.

What an eye opener. Whatever she was getting in those classes was working, and I was so impressed with her results that I began training with Larry myself. The most dramatic changes in Allison's posture occurred as she entered her second year of training, and as the year progressed her improvements accumulated while her spine and neck straightened. According to Allison, this is exactly what Larry had said would occur, that if she remained patient the miracle would happen. I can think of no other instance where an exercise regimen, or any other corrective measure, brought about such dramatic results in repairing someone's posture.

Anne Edwards, M. D., P. C.
Charleston, South Carolina

ANTI - AGING AT ITS BEST

Obstacles to *21st Century Fitness*

In almost any situation people are generally most comfortable with what's familiar or common, and the world of fitness is no different. As I've mentioned throughout the book, one of the leading obstacles to becoming *8 Essential Fit* is the widespread, out-dated image most people have of what it means to be in shape. This image is based on 20th Century aesthetics that glorify muscle mass with little regard for flexibility, agility or the ability to stand tall. Furthermore, the out-dated image is matched with out-dated expectations of the aging process. For some reason few people challenge this notion, and as most move into their later years, they wrongly accept the role of second class citizens, assuming they must ready themselves for losses in appearance and performance. This is just not so, yet these images and expectations have been "bought" by the general public again and again without question.

As a young man, I was a prime example of one who embraced the conventional perception of fitness. Flexibility, agility, standing tall—-none of these were of any concern to me. In fact, during my first visit to the Pilates studio in New York, I was so sure of myself and of my own knowledge of fitness, that I knew there was no way that an old couple and their machines could possibly have anything to offer. "I'll call you for an appointment," I said, but that was only to be polite. I had no intention of learning what seemed to be a strangely curious method of exercise and immediately went back to my glitzy mega-gym where my frozen-in-time ideals were reinforced for years to come.

Roger Servin had long ago instilled in me the correlation between fitness and youth, but as I entered the years I've come to define as the crossover age, I began to realize I was struggling to maintain the body I'd developed as a younger man. There was no sound structure to support my muscle bulk. But this concept was still not clear to me, so, like most people would, I began training harder and harder. I did meet some limited success, and like most, I wrongly believed that as long as I kept working out I could stay young. However, I was confined to my own thinking, and although I had a specific goal, my lack of a clear vision as to how to obtain it and my continued reliance on knowledge of the past only fueled the downturn I was experiencing in my physicality. I define this as a belief in the unknown, and it's another obstacle to becoming *8 Essential Fit*. Today, now that I know differently, it is a fascinating phenomenon to watch in others. People are so quick to embrace a workout regimen, but how many actually consider its long-term effect or its ability to keep them young into their later years? I think it's safe to say not many. This blind abandon is like getting on a plane or a train without knowing your destination.

It's understandable, though. Given the number of magazine and newspaper articles, TV programs, books and day-to-day conversations that broach the subject of fitness, we've been flooded with so much information that most people are under the false impression that we have all the answers. Surely all that's necessary is to try a little of this, a little of that from the "salad bar" of fitness methods and fad diets to achieve our goals. WRONG. This conviction that we already know the answers is perhaps the greatest obstacle in getting the answers. We tend to not ask the all-important questions, "What is fitness?" and "What is it exactly that I want to achieve?" You have to know what you're looking for before you can know if you've found it.

Compounding this belief in the unknown is the popularity of "certified" trainers, but how often do people ask of what their "certification" consists? How and where was it obtained? Will their method provide me with youth in my later years? If so, where's the proof? Can you show me someone over 60 who has followed your training and who possesses the 8 essentials of fitness? If the answer is yes, then these trainers can be wonderful helpers in your effort to become *8 Essential Fit*, but if the answer is no, then such trainers are only another obstacle. The same is true of mega-gyms full of state of the art equipment, any of the latest fitness crazes, celebrity endorsements and the multitude of "experts." Seeing is believing, and unless you have a clear vision of what you're seeking in a fitness program, and unless that vision is backed up with a specific formula of exercise and nutrition you are creating another obstacle for yourself.

As I've already mentioned, most people don't believe that achieving and maintaining the essentials of youth into your later years is possible, that we should quietly accept and expect the traditional aging process. This, coupled with a doom and gloom attitude of, "I might get hit by a bus anyway," is a two-headed obstacle causing generation after generation to grow old before their time. Of course the truth is that you probably won't get hit by a bus, that you'll live a full life, so there is little reason why you shouldn't enjoy those years to their fullest. But this enjoyment won't come from youthful attire, facelifts, liposuction, makeup, hair color or any of the other options available to make us "younger." In fact, while some of these options have merit, they can become obstacles if you rely on them alone. It is only a body built to possess all *8 Essentials of Fitness* that will give us youth in our later years.

Prior to construction, most architects have a clear vision of their structures, and so must we have a clear vision when we design the structure of the body. However, the innovative architects have all had to make a break with the past, and so shall we in overcoming the obstacles of outdated methods and thinking in relation to fitness, methods and thinking that were deeply implanted in my own mind. Just as the architects of the Empire State Building introduced new ideas in design and construction to render the previous ways obsolete, our new understanding of what fitness is will do the same to the common expectations of the unavoidable process of aging.

Assumption

Most people **assume** if we "exercise" and "eat well" we will get "fit."

But do we get specifics? Is there a detailed road map of exercise combined with nutrition that has a beginning and an end result at a given point and time? Are there specific standards and are they complete?

Too long so many have travelled the road to failure continuing to believe the next time will be the answer.

Seeing is believing - understanding the specific goals and the exact method to achieve these goals.

It's about the walk, not the talk. Follow The Winner!

Assumption is the Biggest Obstacle of all!

Retirement Age?

Now you've had a chance to see for yourself that we don't have to age prematurely.

Don't make the mistake I almost made being lured by the conventional wisdom of trying to achieve fitness by "the bits and pieces" of various diets and exercise regimens.

My formula of exercise and nutrition that took a lifetime to develop has given me the youth I longed for in my later years.

It will do the same for you!

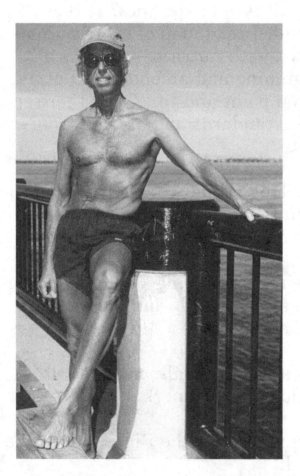

Retirement Age? Never!

21st Century Fitness For Our Children

The former Surgeon General of the United States, Dr. C. Everett Koop, has pointed out that unless Americans significantly alter their eating and exercise habits, virtually everyone in the country will be obese within the first quarter of the 21st Century. The significance of his statement is shattering in regard to the present generation of children. Sadly, as of 2006, this has all come to pass.

Upon entering the 21st Century we've embarked on a new era that promises continuing progress in the fields that affect our day-to-day lives such as telecommunication, science and medicine. Yet with all of our technical advances, the common thinking when applied to fitness and nutrition has remained generally stagnant for over fifty years. For the most part, each generation has reinforced the views and opinions that were handed down from the previous one, and now we are seeing the negative effects in the physical development of our children. It's time for change and choices.

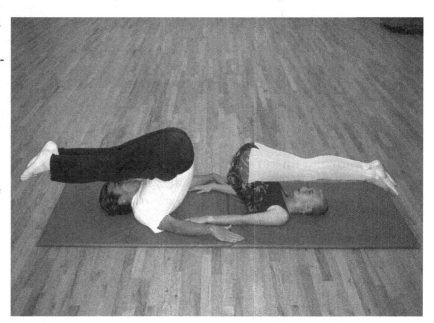

Most fitness programs ignore children, presuming they are more apt to be fit because they lead lives filled with activity. At one time this idea was not off base at all; it was true for just about everyone. The fact is that inactivity has become not only a national trend, but is well on its way to becoming an epidemic - especially in our children. We have only ourselves as parents, the people our kids look to first for example, to blame. We are a nation that celebrates the television and personal computer; often they're the easiest babysitters to find. According to one survey, before a child reaches first grade he or she has watched over 5,000 hours of television, the equivalent of 5-plus hours a day - five-plus hours of inactivity.

In addition to inactivity, poor eating habits are producing an overweight population of children, the likes of which we've never seen. Fast food is a leading culprit, but again we have ourselves to blame because often we provide our children with burgers, fries, sodas and shakes as "rewards." This practice is reinforced by advertising targeted specifically at kids, which creates a cyclical demand. The fast food industry is complemented by the empty-calorie, nutritionally void snack "foods" that are commonly offered, again as "rewards" and "treats." When economic necessity dictates that both parents work, or when there is only one parent in the household, it often becomes easier to "fill 'em up" with snacks and junk food than to prepare nutritionally well balanced meals on a daily basis. While occasional fast food and snacks won't harm children, our tendency as a nation to over-do has not kept the nutritional needs of our children in balance or perspective.

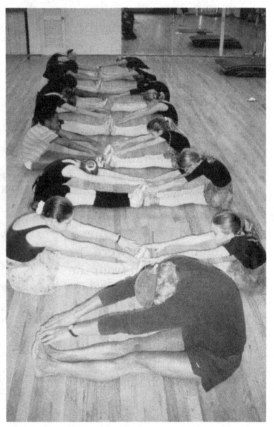

With statistics and wake up calls like the one given by Dr. Koop, the alarm has sounded and the problem identified. A solution? ***21st Century Fitness***. Not only is it a solution, it's an easy solution. Again, it's time for change and choices. We must cultivate and nurture our children's fitness and well-being to combat the sedentary lifestyles we've helped them adopt, and to accomplish this my formula of exercise and nutrition* is ideal.

Having worked with children, I've been amazed with their enthusiasm for the floor work and fill-in exercises. They take to them like they're learning a new sport. However, this sport requires no equipment, can be performed individually or taught to a large group, builds strength and flexibility, hones mental and physical discipline, and, as I've emphasized throughout the book—-it improves posture and alignment. Children are often told to "stand up straight." After all, the first mark of identifying fitness is straightness, but standing tall comes from good posture, and good posture comes from specific exercises and movements that align and position the body so that it stands tall naturally.

* Nutrition with modification—-children require more fat in their diets. Some refined sugar and salt are acceptable, as is the allowance of minimal amounts of refined flour. A childhood without the occasional slice of pizza, birthday cake, or bowl of ice cream would be a sad childhood indeed.

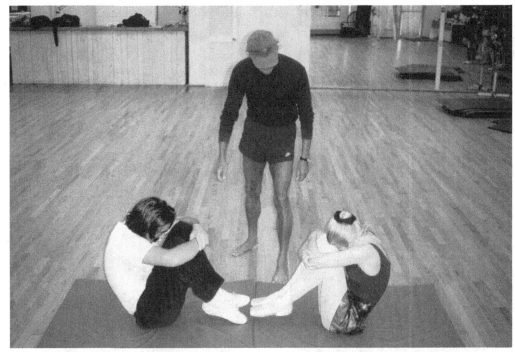

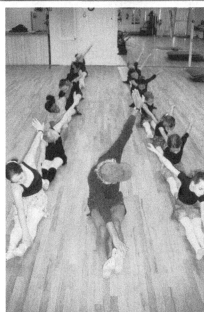 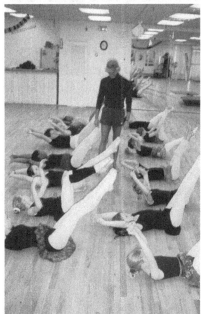

Larry & 8 to 10 year old students

Now is the time to leap into this new dimension of physical fitness. It's time for a new attitude about aging, for change and choices. It's time to take action and turn our expanded vision into reality, starting with our children — in the home, schools and organized groups. Together we can build a nation of children and young adults who are strong, clear-headed, energetic, flexible and who **stand tall** — a nation of families who are *21st Century Fit.*

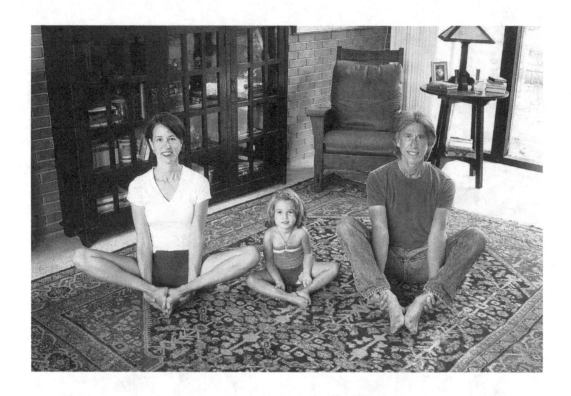

21st Century Fitness, a Family Tradition
Father Larry Nachman, Daughter Beth Nachman Riley,
and Granddaughter Clara Lillian Riley

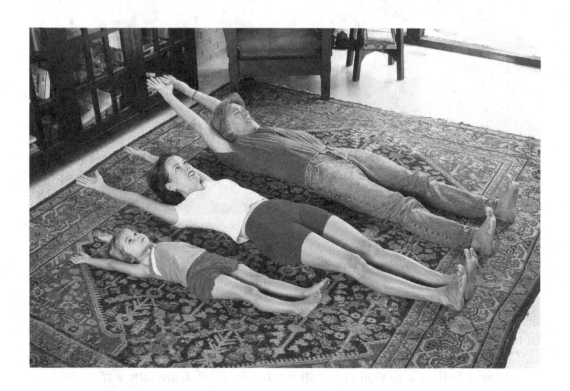

ANTI - AGING AT ITS BEST

21st Century Fitness: MOST DEFINITELY

We can stay young. All you have to do is do it!

Now you know the secret and have seen the **evidence** with your own eyes.

The first proven formula; the ***21st Century Fitness*** formula of exercise and nutrition for long lasting youth really works.

It worked for me.
It worked for my students.
It will work for you.

Join Us. Become a winner!
75 — The New Young is a ***reality!***

Defy Gravity. Build a different kind of body.

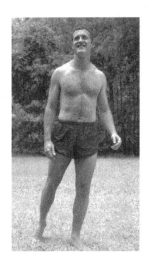
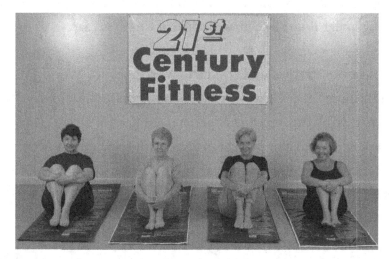
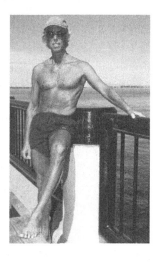
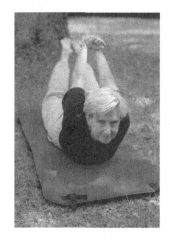
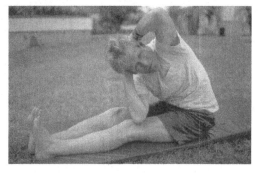

ANTI - AGING AT ITS BEST

Larry Nachman has overcome the traditional aging process and provides visual evidence that people can stay physically young into their 70s. 21st Century Fitness - a unique program that goes beyond Yoga and Pilates provides a new formula of exercise and nutrition. Larry studied under Romana Kryzanowska at the original Pilates Studio in New York for 15 years; and 3 years under Evelyn and Bob Seed at the Bob Seed Studio, also in New York. In addition several years of weight training under Roger Servin, a disciple of Charles Atlas.

Larry lectures, teaches and conducts workshops for World President's Organization; The City of Charleston, South Carolina; Clemson University Athletic Department and has students of all ages (14 to 75) in Charleston; Greenville; and Landrum, South Carolina. In May of 2009, Larry attended his 50th reunion at Tulane University in New Orleans as fit as he was when he graduated in 1959...

A New Standard of Excellence In The World of Fitness.

Nutrition Supplement

Think Mediterranean

I spent two weeks in Venice, Italy in 1977. Given that the three large meals I was served daily were actually sumptuous dining adventures consisting of lots of pasta, veal, chicken, fish, grains, fruits and vegetables, I was certain I would gain at least a few pounds over the course of my stay. When I returned to New York I'd lost three pounds.

I couldn't get over it. I ate as well or better than I ever had in my life, and yet my weight actually dropped. It was then I realized that the combinations of food that the Mediterranean people had developed over thousands of years offered more than merely delicious meals. These foods and their combinations were balanced to my physical needs, and they provided me not only with sustenance, but mental gratification from knowing I was treating my body well. I then promised myself, to adopt this wonderful cuisine.

While this book is not designed to provide recipes, here are some standouts from my experience that I believe will whet your appetites.

Tomato & Bread Salad with Basil and Red Onion
(serves 6 for appetizers)

1/3 cup red wine vinegar
8 oz. stale whole grain bread
   cut into 2" pieces
2 lbs. Ripe plum tomatoes
   coarsely chopped (about 5 cups)

1/2 cup extra-virgin olive oil
8 cups cold water
1 small red onion
1 cup loosely packed fresh
   basil leaves, torn into bite-
   size pieces

Pour vinegar into small bowl. Gradually whisk in oil. Season vinaigrette to taste with salt and pepper.

Place bread in large bowl. Pour in enough cold water (about 8 cups) to cover bread. Soak 5 minutes and drain well. Squeeze bread to remove as much liquid as possible. Coarsely crumble bread into same bowl. Add tomatoes, onion and basil. Toss with enough vinaigrette to coat. Season salad with salt and pepper. (Can be made 8 hours ahead. Cover and refrigerate. Let stand 1 hour at room temperature before serving.)

Classic Tuscan Flatbread

1 cup lukewarm water (90-100 degrees F.)
2 1/4 oz. packages dry yeast or
   2 .6 oz. packages fresh yeast, crumbled
2 1/2 cups (about) all-purpose whole grain flour
4 tbsp. extra virgin olive oil
1 tbsp. coarse sea salt

Pour 1 cup lukewarm water into small bowl; sprinkle with yeast. Let stand until yeast dissolves, about 10 minutes.

Place 2 cups flour in large bowl. Make well in center of flour. Pour yeast mixture into well. Using fork, stir until dough comes together. Knead into bowl, adding enough flour, 1/4 cup at a time, to form slightly sticky dough. Transfer to floured work surface. Knead until dough is smooth and elastic, about 10 minutes. Coat bowl with 1 tbsp. oil. Add dough, turn to coat. Cover bowl with plastic wrap. Let stand in warm, draft-free area until doubled, about 1 hour and 15 minutes.

Brush 11" diameter tart pan with removable bottom or baking sheet with 1 tbsp. extra virgin olive oil. Punch down dough. Turn out onto whole grain floured work surface and shape into 11" round. Transfer dough to prepared tart pan or baking sheet. Cover loosely with plastic. Let rise until dough is almost doubled, about 30 minutes.

Preheat oven to 400 degrees F. Press fingertips into dough, creating indentations. Brush with remaining 2 tbsp. oil. Sprinkle with salt. Bake until golden, about 28 minutes. Cool bread in pan on rack 10 minutes. Remove bread from pan and let cool completely.

Faro Salad with Peas, Favas, Arugula and Tomatoes
(8 entree servings)

6 cups water	2 cups faro or wheat berries
5 tbsp. olive oil	2 1/2 tbsp. red wine vinegar
1 cup shelled fresh fava beans	1 cup shelled fresh or frozen peas
or frozen baby lima beans	2 cups fresh arugula leaves,
3 plum tomatoes, seeded,	halved
finely chopped	Additional arugula leaves

Combine 6 cups water and faro in medium saucepan. Bring to boil. Reduce heat to medium. Cover partially; simmer until faro is tender, about 20 minutes. (About 45 minutes for wheat berries). Drain well.

Whisk oil and vinegar in large bowl. Season with salt. Add faro and toss. Let cool. Meanwhile, cook favas in pot of boiling salted water for 3 minutes. Add peas and cook until just tender, about 1 minute longer. Drain. Cool in bowl of ice water and drain. Add favas and peas to faro. (Can be made 4 hours ahead, then covered and chilled.)

Add arugula and tomatoes to faro mixture and toss. Season generously with salt, and spoon salad onto platter. Garnish with additional arugula.

White Beans with Sage and Olive Oil
(6 side dish servings)

1 lb. dried Great Northern beans	6 cups cold water
1/4 cup extra virgin olive oil	1 1/2 tbsp. chopped fresh sage
1 large garlic clove, minced	Additional olive oil

Place beans in large saucepan. Add enough cold water to cover by 3", and let soak overnight.

Drain beans and return to pan. Add 6 cups cold water, 1/4 cup oil, chopped sage and garlic. Bring to boil. Reduce heat to medium-low. Cover partially and simmer until beans are just tender, stirring occasionally, about 45 minutes. Season with salt and pepper. (Can be made 1 day ahead. After cooling, cover and keep chilled. Re-warm before continuing.)

Using slotted spoon, transfer beans to bowl. Top with more oil.

Linguine with Shellfish Sauce
(4-6 entree servings)

6 tbsp. extra virgin olive oil	2 garlic cloves, minced
3/4 tsp. Dried crushed red pepper	12 oz. cleaned squid, bodies cut
1 1/4 cups dry white wine	into 1/2" wide rings. Tentacles
1 28 oz. can Italian style tomatoes	left whole.
1/4 cup water	2 lbs. Small littleneck clams,
2 tsp. Tomato paste	scrubbed
1 lb. mussels, scrubbed, debearded	8 oz. Uncooked large shrimp,
1 10 oz. uncooked lobster tailed,	peeled, deveined
shelled, meat cut into 1" pieces	4 oz. bay scallops
3 tbsp. chopped fresh Italian	1 lb. linguine
parsley	

Heat 3 tbsp. oil in large skillet over medium heat. Add garlic and crushed red pepper; stir 1 minute. Add squid; sauté just until opaque, about 3 minutes. Add wine; simmer until liquid is reduced by half, about 20 minutes.

Anti - Aging at its best

Add tomatoes with juices and tomato paste. Bring to simmer, breaking up tomatoes. Cover and simmer over low heat 40 minutes.

Bring 1/4 cup water to boil in another large skillet over high heat. Add clams and mussels. Cover, cook until shells open, about 6 minutes (discard any clams or mussels that do not open). Transfer shellfish to colander set over medium bowl and drain.

Strain juices from skillet and medium bowl through fine sieve into tomato sauce. Simmer sauce uncovered until slightly thickened, about 10 minutes. Add lobster, shrimp and scallops. Simmer 2 minutes. Add clams and mussels from colander. Simmer 1 minute longer. Stir in remaining 2 tbsp. oil and parsley. Season with salt and pepper.

Meanwhile you should have cooked linguine in large pot of boiling salted water until just tender but still firm to bite. Drain and return to pot. Add shellfish and toss to coat.

Shrimp in Garlic Sauce

1/3 cup olive oil	4 cloves garlic, sliced
2 small red chili peppers	3/4 lb. small shrimp, peeled
1 tablespoon minced parsley	A little lemon juice (optional)

Heat the oil and add the garlic and chili peppers. When garlic begins to turn golden, add shrimp and salt. Cook shrimp about 1 minute. Sprinkle with parsley and lemon juice. Serve with bread.

Piquillo Toasts

Top toasted baguette slices with diced piquillo peppers (these can be found at specialty food stores or replaced with roasted red peppers). Sauté sliced garlic in olive oil, add lemon juice and drizzle over peppers. Garnish with chopped parsley.

Cerviche

2 lbs. Scallops	4 cups water
2 cups fresh lime juice	1 large onion, chopped
2 tablespoons tamari or light soy sauce	2 large cucumbers, peeled, seeded and cut into half moons
1 yellow pepper, chopped	1 bunch fresh dill, chopped
salt and pepper to taste	

Combine water, lime juice, onion and soy sauce to make a marinade. Add the scallops and refrigerate for about 30 minutes. Add the cucumbers, pepper, dill and salt and pepper and serve.

Lentil Feta Salad
(4-6 entree or side servings)

1 cup beluga lentils or French green lentils, rinsed

2 stalks celery, finely chopped

1 small red pepper, roasted, peeled and finely diced

1 tbsp. finely chopped rosemary

2 tbsp. extra virgin olive oil

4 oz. feta cheese (about 1 cup) coarsely crumbled, salt and peppered to taste

2 cloves garlic, halved lengthwise

1 bay leaf

1 small red onion, diced

1 cup fresh flat-leaf parsley, finely chopped

1/3 cup freshly squeezed lemon juice

3 heads baby lettuce, for garnish

1 small cucumber, peeled, seeded and cut into 1/8" slices

Bring medium saucepan of water to boil. Add lentils, garlic and bay leaf. Simmer for 20 minutes, or until lentils are tender. Drain, and rinse lentils under cold water. Discard garlic and bay leaf. In a large bowl combine lentils, celery, onion, pepper, parsley and rosemary.

In a small bowl whisk together lemon juice and olive oil. Drizzle over lentil mixture, add feta and stir gently to incorporate.

While the spotlight here has been on the Mediterranean/Tuscan style of food choices and preparation, the idea behind these applies to practically any of the hundreds of cuisines of the world. The principles and elements, once understood, provide a freedom of choice to appease the particular tastes and cravings of almost anyone.

The following are recipes from other cuisines.

Cassoulet
(Makes 8 servings)

1 1/4 pounds, skinless chicken breast or 1 can pork tenderloin,*
    cut into 3/4 inch pieces

12 ounces smoked sausage (97 % fat free),
    cut into 1/2 inch slices

1 tablespoon olive oil

1 1/2 cups chopped onion

1 cup chopped red bell pepper

4 to 6 teaspoons minced garlic, to taste

4 (5 ounce) cans Great Northern beans, rinsed and drained;
    or 2 cups dry-packaged Great Northern beans, cooked

1 (14 1/2 ounce) can diced tomatoes with roasted garlic

1 teaspoon dried thyme leaves
1 3/4 cups fat-free, reduced-sodium chicken broth
Salt and pepper, to taste
2 1/2 cups fresh whole-wheat or whole grain bread crumbs

Sauté chicken or pork and sausage in oil in Dutch oven until lightly brown, 8-10 minutes. Add onion, bell pepper and 3 to 5 teaspoons garlic, to taste; cook over medium heat 5 minutes. Stir in beans, tomatoes, thyme and chicken broth; season to taste with salt and pepper.

Combine bread crumbs and remaining garlic; sprinkle over top of bean mixture. Bake, uncovered at 350 degrees until crumbs are browned and beans are thickened, about 1 1/2 hours.

Roasted Eggplant Caesar Salad
(serves 8)

2 Med. Eggplants cubed
1 Med. Red pepper julienned
1/2 lb. Silken tofu
4 anchovy fillets
2 tbsp. Fresh lemon juice
4 tsp. Olive oil
**1/3 cup grated Parmesan cheese

2 Red Onions julienned
1 Med. Yellow bell pepper
   julienned
2 tbsp. Dijon mustard
4 tsp. Garlic paste
Salt and pepper

*Occasional lean pork is okay.
** A small amount of cheese as a garnish is okay.

Preheat oven to 325 Degrees F. Place vegetables on a baking sheet and roast until tender, about 25 minutes. Set aside. In a food processor, combine the tofu, anchovies, mustard, lemon juice, garlic paste and olive oil. Season with salt and pepper. Fold into roasted vegetables. Serve sprinkled with grated Parmesan cheese.

Per serving: 122 calories; 5 g. fat; 5 mg cholesterol; 253 mg. Sodium.

Grilled Vegetable "Lasagna" with Herbed
Tofu and Red Pepper Sauce
(serves 8)

1 medium onion
2 tsp. Extra Virgin Olive oil
3 cups low-sodium fat free
   vegetable broth
1 medium yellow squash

2 cloves garlic
1 large eggplant
1 tbsp. chopped cilantro
1 13 oz. Jar roasted red
   peppers, drained

1 medium zucchini
1 medium butternut squash
    (store-bought is fine)
1 lb. Soft tofu
1/2 cup mixed fresh herbs

2 cups balsamic vinegarette
8 medium Portobello mushrooms
1 cup dried breadcrumbs
Salt and pepper

To make the red pepper sauce, combine the onion, garlic and oil in a medium saucepan and sauté over medium-high heat until tender but not browned. Add the peppers and broth; heat to boiling. Reduce heat to low and simmer, 10 minutes. Remove from heat and mix in a food processor until smooth. Strain through a sieve into a clean saucepan. Stir in the cilantro. Add salt and pepper to taste. Keep warm.

Cut eggplant into eight slices. Cut the zucchini and yellow squash diagonally into eight slices, peel butternut squash neck and cut into eight slices. Remove stems from mushrooms. Put in a bowl, add the vinaigrette and marinate 20 minutes.

Light grill or heat broiler. Remove vegetables from marinade and cook, about 5 minutes, turning once.

In a blender or food processor, combine tofu, breadcrumbs and herbs. Pulse until smooth. Blend in salt and pepper to taste. Put in a microwave-safe bowl, cover and cook on high power about 1 minute. Alternately, put tofu mixture in double-boiler top over hot water and heat gently, stirring frequently until warm, about 10 min.

To serve, put one mushroom on each of eight plates, spread with some of the herbed tofu. Top with a slice of another vegetable and more tofu. Repeat using one of each kind of vegetable, sandwiching some tofu between for each serving. Pour about 1/2 cup of sauce around each lasagna.

Per serving: 264 Calories; 8 g. fat; 0 mg. cholesterol; 957 mg. sodium.

Chicken and Shrimp Gumbo
(Serves 6-8)

1 cup whole grain flour
1/4 lb. Chicken or turkey
    sausage, diced
1 medium sweet pepper,
    seeded half , cubed
4 scallions, sliced
1 medium jalapeno, mince
1 28 oz. can sliced tomatoes
2 tsp. dried parsley
1 tsp. dried thyme
1 tsp. dried basil
1/2 tsp. onion powder
2 cups cooked millet
1 tsp. gumbo fillet

1 tsp. Extra Virgin Olive oil
1 boneless, skinless chicken
    breast half cubed
2 celery stalks, diced
1 medium onion, diced
2 large garlic cloves minced
1 1/2 cups sliced fresh okra
4 cups low-sodium fat free
    chicken or vegetable stock
1 tsp. dried oregano
1 bay leaf
8 large shrimp, peeled
    and deveined

ANTI - AGING AT ITS BEST

Heat oven to 350° F. Put flour on a baking sheet and toast in the oven, stirring frequently, until well browned, about 30 minutes.

Heat the oil in a large saucepan over medium heat and sauté the sausage and chicken breast until no longer pink. Add the pepper, celery, onion, scallions, garlic, jalapeno and okra. Cook over medium heat until onion is translucent. Stir the flour into the pot with the chicken and vegetables and stir until evenly coated. Add the stock, tomatoes and their liquid, herbs and onion powder. Simmer 30 minutes, stirring occasionally.

Turkey Tortilla Roll
(Serves 2)

1 tsp. garlic	1 tsp. each of oregano, thyme,
1/8 tsp. each of salt and	and sage, mixed
pepper mixed	8 oz. skinless turkey breast
1 tsp. Extra Virgin Olive oil	(pound thin)
1/2 tsp. garlic	4 oz. julienne mixed vegetables
sea salt and pepper to taste	(carrot, zucchini, yellow
10" whole grain flour tortilla	squash and red cabbage)

Marinate the turkey breast with the garlic, oregano, thyme and sage for a minimum of one hour, then grill or sauté.

Sauté mixed vegetables with garlic in olive oil, season with salt and pepper, and let cool.

Arrange cooked julienne vegetables in the center of the tortilla. Add grilled turkey breast sliced 1/4" thick on top of vegetables. Season with a touch of salt and pepper, roll up the tortilla.

Heat in microwave for 40 seconds.
Serve with your favorite bean dish for good food combining.

Per Serving: 287 Calories, 9 g. Total Fat, 88 mg. Cholesterol, 629 mg. Sodium, 45 g. Carbohydrates, 45 g. Protein.

Stir Fry Sauce with Vegetables
(Servings 4 - 6)

1/2 cup sherry or Marsala wine	3 oz. fresh ginger, sliced
1 tbsp. shallots, chopped	1 tbsp. garlic, chopped
1 cup mirin	3/4 cup wheat-free tamari
2 cups filtered water	2 tbsp. arrow root powder
toasted sesame seeds (optional)	(mixed with 2 tbsp.
	filtered water)

Deglaze sherry/Marsala wine with ginger, shallots, and garlic by half. Add mirin, tamari, and filtered water. Let boil for 5 minutes.

Add arrow root powdered mix and simmer for 5 minutes. Sauté 1 1/2 cups of your favorite seasonal vegetables in 4 oz. of Stir Fry Sauce.

Serve with 4 oz. of brown rice, season with salt and pepper. Sprinkle with toasted sesame seeds if desired.

Per Serving: 96 Calories, 0 g. Total Fat, 0 mg. Cholesterol, 2,015 mg. Sodium, 9 g. Carbohydrate, 4 g. Protein.

Chili-Seared Shrimp Marinade
(Servings: 9 servings of 4 shrimp each)

36 medium shrimp, peeled and cleaned
1 1/2 oz. tamari
2 tbsp. chili garlic paste
1 tbsp. Extra Virgin olive oil

2 oz. tomato paste
1 1/2 tsp. ground coriander seed
1 oz. mirin
1 tbsp. lemon juice
1 1/2 tbsp. ancho chili powder (mild chili can be substituted for any chili powder)

Whisk all ingredients together.
Add Shrimp, refrigerate a minimum of 6 hours, up to 26 hours.
Sear in hot nonstick pan rubbed with olive oil, one minute on each side.
Serve on baked whole grain tortilla chips with a dollop of guacamole and seared shrimp set on top.

Per Serving: 141 Calories, 6 g. Total Fat, 98 mg. Cholesterol, 851 mg. Sodium, 7 g. Carbohydrate, 15 g. Protein.

Scotch Broth

6 cups chicken broth, fat free, low sodium
Extra Virgin Olive oil
To Taste > Barley, carrots and turnips
Garlic (1 clove)
6 cups cabbage
1 onion
1 cup skinless chopped chicken

Gazpacho Soup

2 medium size cucumbers
1 bunch shallots
2 whole tomatoes
1 medium size green tomatoes
2 cloves garlic
1 tablespoon chopped parsley
2 small cans tomato juice
2 cups beef bouillon
1 tablespoon apple cider vinegar
2 tablespoons worcestershire sauce
1/2 teaspoon tabasco

Finely chop an mix cucumber, tomatoes, shallots, green pepper, parsley and garlic. Add tomato juice, vinegar, bouillon, tabasco, and worcestershire sauce. Chill and serve. (Serves 4)

Shrimp Remoulade

3/4 cup minced parsley
3/4 cup minced shallots
3/4 cup minced celery
3/4 cup minced dill pickle
1 tablespoon minced garlic
1 3/4 cup creole hot mustard
3 tablespoons horseradish
1/2 cup apple cider vinegar
1/4 cup extra virgin olive oil

Mix all ingredients together and chill. The longer it stands, the better the taste. Add the cooked shrimp and eat up.

Red beans and Rice

2 cups kidney beans
1/2 cup chopped white onion
1/2 cup chopped shallots
1/2 teaspoon minced garlic
1/4 cup extra virgin olive oil
1/4 cup fat free sausage
1/4 cup skinless chicken
3 cups water
1 teaspoon salt
1/2 teaspoon black pepper

Soak beans overnight. Drain. In large saucepan saute onions, shallots and garlic in olive oil until tender. Add sausage and chicken and continue cooking until lightly browned. Add drained kidney beans and remaining ingredients. Cook slowly 45 minutes to one hour if needed. Serve with brown rice. tabasco as desired.

Creole Jambalaya

1 cup chopped white onion
1/2 cup chopped green pepper
1/2 cup chopped celery
1 teaspoon minced garlic
1/2 cup extra virgin olive oil
1 cup raw shrimp
1 cup raw oysters
2 cups whole tomatoes
1 cup water
1 bay leaf
1/2 teaspoon salt
1/4 teaspoon cayenne
1 cup raw brown rice

In large saucepan saute onion, green peppers, celery and garlic in olive oil until tender. Add shrimp and oysters, cook five minutes. Add remaining ingredients except rice and cook over low heat 10 to 15 minutes more. Add rice, stir and cover tightly. Cook 25 to 30 minutes over low heat until rice is done. (4 servings)

White Bean Salad With Shrimp and Asparagus

Warm vinaigrette wilts fresh spinach. This salad is best eaten immediately after tossing.

2 cups (1-inch) sliced asparagus (about 1/2 pound)
3/4 pound medium shrimp, peeled and deveined
1/2 teaspoon freshly ground black pepper, divided
1/4 teaspoon salt, divided
1 teaspoon virgin olive oil
2 cups torn spinach
1 (19 oz.) can cannelli beans, drained and rinsed
3 turkey bacon slices (fat free)
1/2 cup chopped Vidalia green onions
1 garlic clove, minced
1/4 cup fat-free, no sodium chicken broth
1 tablespoon chopped fresh parsley
2 tablespoons fresh lemon juice
1 tablespoon cider vinegar

Directions:
Steam asparagus, covered, 3 minutes. Drain and rinse with cold water. Sprinkle shrimp with 1/8 teaspoon pepper and 1/8 teaspoon salt; toss well. Heat oil in a medium nonstick skillet over medium-high heat. Add shrimp; saute' 4 minutes. Remove from pan; place in a large bowl. Add asparagus, spinach, and beans to shrimp; toss well. Add turkey bacon to pan; cook over medium heat until crisp. Remove turkey bacon from pan. Crumble reserve teaspoon drippings. Cook onions & garlic until soft. Remove from heat, add remaining ingredients, drizzle over salad.

Pancakes: A Great Sunday Breakfast

- multi-grain pancake mix
- raw oats
- banana
- 2 egg whites
- 1/2 teaspoon extra virgin olive oil
- Ginger
- vanilla to taste
- water as needed
- 3 tablespoons raw wheat germ

Spray pan with PAM fat free 100% virgin olive oil cooking spray. Use raw honey as syrup. (Spread lightly over pancakes.)

GET THE IDEA?

HAVE FUN!
and
GOOD LUCK!

Acknowledgements

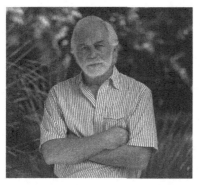

To **David Grant** of Charleston, South Carolina for his help in getting this project off the ground. His support was invaluable.

The author wishes to thank the following people for their assistance in writing this book: Hartwell Littlejohn, Ashley Adams, Richard Dowell, and Kimberley Westbury.

Lynne Nachman and Sheila Grant for their patience and support.

A special thanks to my students who modeled in the book and for writing their stories.

Also to Paula Netzky Spiegel, the late Geraldine Delaney and the staff at Little Hill/Alina Lodge.

To Brad Forth for front and back cover photographs.
To Owen Riley, Jr. — a special thanks for your patience and for the majority of photographs in this book.

Note: None of the photographs of Larry were altered or modified to enhance his physique or appearance.

In June of 2001, my brother-in-law, Dr. Robert Kramer of Dallas, Texas, invited me to join him for lunch with Stanley Marcus, chairman emeritus of Neiman Marcus. While driving to the restaurant, we talked about my theories on fitness. To my amazement, at age 96, Stanley said he regretted that he had not understood how important posture was to fitness and that he had not worked on it early in life.

At this time I had been in a "lounging mode" and not working on my book. This comment, at this exact moment in time, hit me between the eyes. It re-ignited my fire to get on with 21st Century Fitness.

The late Stanley Marcus, always one to zero in on the world of fashion and retail, had again zeroed in on the world of fitness.

Notice to Readers

It is recommended that you consult your Doctor if you suffer from any health problems or special conditions before starting the 21st Century Fitness Formula of exercise and Nutrition.

1st Edition, 21st Century Fitness. April 2002
Published April 2002
By
21st Century Enterprises in Charleston, South Carolina
Web site: www.21stCenturyFitness.com
email: Larry@21stCenturyFitness.com

2nd Edition, 21st Century Fitness: 70 The New Young. January 2007

3rd Edition, 21st Century Fitness: Beyond Yoga...Beyond Pilates. November 2013

© Copyright 2002 21st Century Enterprises. All rights reserved.
Library of Congress
TUx 843-195

US Trademark Registration No. 2352176 for : *21st Century Fitness*®

No part of this publication, except for short excerpts for review purposes, may be reproduced in any form (including photocopying or storage in any medium by electronic means) without the written prior consent of the author.

Printed in the United States of America.

National Library of Canada Cataloguing in Publication

Nachman, Larry, 1937-
21st century fitness : a formula of exercise and nutrition for staying young
Larry Nachman and David Grant.
ISBN 1-55395-133-6
1. Exercise. 2. Nutrition. I. Grant, David II. Title.
III. Title: Twenty-first century fitness.
RA781.N32 2002   613.7   C2002-904636-X

Printed in the United States
By Bookmasters